The Roots of Natural Mothering

The Roots of Natural Mothering--

Through the Seasons of Pregnancy,
Journey of Birth,
And Motherbaby Moon Time

Janice Marsh-Prelesnik

© Allison McKenna

Mother Muse Publishing
Galesburg, Michigan

Mother Muse Publishing

12901 Fort Custer Drive

Galesburg, MI 49053

(269) 665-7797

http://www.creativebirthingarts.com

ISBN 0-9764712-0-5

Printing by Fidlar/Doubleday, Kalamazoo, MI

Photos © 2004 by Janice Marsh-Prelesnik

Cover design by Allison McKenna

Dedication

This book is dedicated to my daughter, Heather, and to my sons, Jarek, Garth, and Jesse, their future partners, and all of the other young people of the world who will bring forth future generations. May you care for your babies and yourselves gently, while being embraced in the gifts of natural processes and cared for by Mother Earth.

Acknowledgements

With deep gratitude I would like to first thank the divine spirit for guiding me through this project.

To my family—lifetime partner Lee, and children Heather, Jarek, Garth, and Jesse, thanks from the bottom of my heart for your patience. I know, Lee, that my "clutter bombs" of books and papers everywhere drive you crazy. Thank you for once again being patient with me. I appreciate that you all cared for me when my mind was deep in thought and slow to switch to the reality and needs of moment. I love you all with every cell in my body.

To Mom and Grandma—though you both have parted from this earth in body form, I know the two of you are always with me buried deep in my every cell. Every day I think about how you nurtured me and taught me about true gutsy, unconditional, and everlasting love.

A big hug and thank you goes to the women that I interviewed. Alison, Kim, Linda, Lorelei, Lorene, Marisol, and Ruth Anne; I admire your courage for listening to your intuitive voice and mothering in a way that you know is right for you.

To Laurie, Lee, and Iris Arboreal of Eater's Guild Organic Farm—a big thank you for offering your front porch to me while I was writing over the summer. Thank you for the copious amount of organic veggies, which I munched on while writing. You, my friends, are midwives of Mother Earth.

To Sara Wickham—never could there be a more supportive friend. Thank you for your encouragement and good faith in my work.

Rebecca Barnebey, my advisor from Goddard College, has been invaluable as a guide and writing mentor for this project. Thank you, Rebecca, for gently and patiently encouraging me to bring forth this work.

A big thanks goes to Suzanne Richman, director of the Health Arts and Sciences program at Goddard College. Without her vision and wisdom I may never have had the perseverance to finish this book.

In between changing diapers, final exams, and work, my friends, Lisa Thorne and Allison McKenna, edited and formatted this book for me. Thank you both for listening to me when I ranted about my lack of computer skills, and thanks for finding time to be a part of this project.

To my baby crone midwife friends—thanks for all of the stories and sharing throughout the years. I have such a deep love and respect for all of you. You are amazing women.

And last, but certainly not least, thank you to all of the women who have asked me to attend them as their midwife. I consider it a great honor. I have learned so much about life from all of you.

TABLE OF CONTENTS

Introduction

The natural process of the growth of a new baby, from conception to birth, and the care of the motherbaby does not need to be considered a medical event, but rather, a holy, sacred time in the lives of a new family. It is my deep longing that the women of the world and their families come to understand that the seasons of pregnancy, journey of birth, and motherbaby moon time, are indeed profoundly spiritual and sacred moments in time. Experiencing this natural process to the fullest, with spiritual awareness, brings an added depth and understanding to a new mother, and influences her mothering, for the rest of her life.

Attitudes and beliefs will affect how a woman births and how she cares for her baby. Giving this experience over to the medical care industry effects how a woman feels about herself both as a woman, and as a mother. The way a mother birthed and cared for baby will be deeply embedded in that child's way of being. Women are born with the inborn ability to grow, birth, and care for their babies. My dream is that women do trust, or learn to trust and believe in, the great design of what nature has intended.

Women, by being born women, intuitively know how to do this work. Natural mothers, and the midwives that attend them, know and trust the entire process. Judy Luce, a midwife from Vermont, writes on this idea in an article, *The Knowing Body and Remembering Heart,*

> A midwife assures a woman that she does "know" how to give birth; it is genetically encoded in each of her cells. It is a "memory" that came through her mother and her mother's mother and before; the umbilical cord of knowledge and inspiration coils back in time and into the future in the birth of our daughters (Luce, 2004, p.19).

My fear is that future generations of women could forget how to be natural mothers if their mothers before them had given themselves over to the medical world. The life we live becomes encoded in the deepest parts of our being. In the words of medical intuitive and author Caroline Myss, "Our biography becomes our biology" (Myss, 2004, p.40).

We must carefully consider what is lost when mothers give themselves and their babies to the Western medical way of thinking. In much of the United States the cesarean rate is 27% of all births. The epidural rates are skyrocketing. We are in danger of forgetting how to birth our own babies, simply because we are being convinced that we aren't able to do it, or that we shouldn't want to fully experience these sacred seasons of our lives as mothers.

Our culture has a campaign to "Say No to Drugs." And yet, a majority of the babies are born with drugs flowing through their bodies. Is there any wonder that there are many health issues with our children when they were bottle fed, vaccinated, and fed a less than optimally nutritious diet? Is there any wonder that many children lack emotional health when they were not held closely to their mothers as infants so that their baby language could be listened to in a timely fashion?

When a mother chooses to become a natural mother she chooses to connect, or reconnect, with biological order. The wisdom of nature and natural process are her guides. This ancient knowledge comes to a natural mother through her intuition.

As you read through this book you won't find information concerning the myriad of medical tests and interventions that are offered to women and their babies. Indeed, the philosophy of natural mothering assumes that the natural processes will provide until shown otherwise. Occasionally, we do need to look towards medicine for support. At these times, we look to the wisdom of our intuitive voice to guide us to appropriate care. The focus will be on staying healthy, both emotionally and physically, and looking inwards to the deeper self.

This book is written in two sections. The first section explores natural mothering through the seasons of pregnancy, journey of birth and motherbaby moon time, and the second section focuses on staying healthy through the seasons.

Whether the ideas in this book are new to you or you are already familiar with this mothering lifestyle, please, walk with me now through a journey of the roots of natural mothering.

Section One:

Journey Through the Seasons

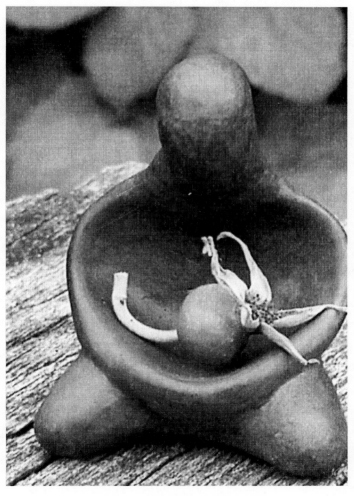

© Janice Marsh-Prelesnik

~One~

The Roots of Natural Mothering

In this book we will explore natural mothering through the seasons of pregnancy. Trusting the natural process of growing and birthing your baby, relying on your intuition as a valid way of knowing, living an earth-centered life style, and holistic health care; these will be your guides as you journey through the exciting adventure of creating a new being.

Recognizing that we are all unique individuals, a natural mother will gather resources and then make decisions based on what is right for her unique motherbaby (meaning unity of mother and baby) bond. A natural mother creates her own path; a path that is less followed and sometimes unfamiliar to others. If you choose this mothering style it may at times feel as though the path is rocky and uphill. You may not have the support of family and friends, as natural mothering as a whole is not yet generally accepted or understood in the culture we live in. You must be strong, however, and learn to stand on your own two feet. Creating this style of mothering paves the way for future mothers.

Recently, I was the midwife for a young woman who herself was born at home, extensively breastfed, carried almost constantly as an infant, and slept with her parents. She so enjoyed how she was raised that she didn't have to agonize over how she would birth and raise her baby. Natural mothering had been taught to her. How beautiful it was that she was able to follow a path where the brambles had been cleared for her. Her family wholeheartedly accepted her choices.

While the path may not always be cleared for all women it is more common now for mothers to practice this mothering style. It certainly makes the process of decision making easier when you know others who have made similar decisions.

In general the guiding principles of natural mothering are:

- ♥ Trusting in natural process
- ♥ Natural childbirth
- ♥ Intuition as guide
- ♥ Holistic natural health care
- ♥ Whole foods diet
- ♥ A birth assistant who follows the holistic model of care
- ♥ No separation of motherbaby at birth

- ♥ Breastfeeding
- ♥ Attachment parenting (staying close to your baby at all times)
- ♥ Following the natural rhythms of baby

As mentioned, these are guiding ideals. The options are endless as you weave the tapestry of your mothering life. As Lorene, a mother of four, says, *"You don't have to do all of these things, but once you get started on one, the rest often seem to follow. It has a snowball effect."*

Each of these principles will be explored in depth in this book. Can one be a natural mother and not follow all of the aspects of natural mothering? Yes, of course. Women need to stand with respect and understanding for each other that we all make our own decisions based on what is right for ourselves and our family. It is absolutely imperative that we support one another for every choice that is made. Sometimes the reality of life doesn't support our wish to live an ideal. Or perhaps our inner self isn't yet ready to make a lifestyle change. Given time, attitudes and values can, and do, transform.

A natural mother is a wise woman and knows that she must always center on the uniqueness of each situation. Like a gentle breeze she flows with the moment. She knows herself and her baby better than anyone else and makes her decisions based on the needs of the moment. She listens to her own heart and follows what she needs to keep herself in balance. The old saying, "If Mama ain't happy, ain't nobody happy," seems a little extreme, but it is true. A natural mother cares for herself so that she can care for others.

In this book you will read many quotes and ideas from experienced mothers. Their words have been italicized so that they may be easily identified. I interviewed seven women, whom are the mothers of a total of 35 children, ranging in ages from six months to twenty-three years.

These words are their definitions of natural mothering:

Natural mothering is following your instincts and doing what innately feels right.

❂

I would say that natural mothering is mothering with the intentions of following the rhythms of the family as a whole.

❂

Intuitive, I would say first of all; intuitive and responsive. I would also say "down to earth," and that means practical.

✪

It means raising them in a way that is comfortable for me. Raising them myself, and thinking through what would work the best for my family and for each child. Not relying on outside help.

✪

Mothering the way that comes natural to you. So mothering naturally would be mothering how my heart tells me to do things rather than what society tells me to do.

✪

Natural mothering means trusting and following the rhythms of natural process.

✪

Natural mothering is following the heart rather than the head.

✪

Natural mothering is attachment parenting. It is a lifestyle. Ideally, that means that you give birth naturally, breastfeed, sleep with your baby, eat whole foods, and carry your baby with you throughout the day.

✪

Natural mothering is a spiritual path. It means staying connected with family on a deep level and making that your top priority.

✪

Since the beginning of human kind the natural mother has laid the foundation for the nurturing of our species. She has birthed her infant naturally, held her baby close, and nourished her baby at her breast.

The prolonged mother-child bond was the root of human sociability, and the nurturing response of the mother to her child became a model for human interaction. It prepared both female and male children to live in a world where attachment to, caring about, and collaboration with other humans was natural to life (Kimmel, 2003, p.2).

Feminine wisdom and divine love are the guiding lights. This wisdom is the collective voice of all mothers: ancient and present. The following poem speaks of the call to eternal voices to guide us along.

Eternal Voices

Spirit voices—
Eternal Mother,
Please… share your wisdom and
Guide me on my way.

Ancient voices—
Mothers before me,
Send your divine light,
To my wondering soul.

Teach me stillness,
Show me the way.
The journey of forever,
Is in the ancient past.

Your voyage of long ago,
Has become,
My voyage of this moment,
In mystical time.

The ways of nurturing,
And mothering this new life,
Are revealed to me,
Through your guidance.

With gratitude,
I bow down before you.
I honor your wisdom,
Of bringing forth new life.

Spirit voices—
Eternal Mother,
Please… share your wisdom,
And guide me on my way.

Ancient voices—
Mothers before me.
Send your divine light,
To my wondering soul.

©Janice Marsh-Prelesnik, 2004

I offer this book to you in the spirit of sharing wisdom from my twenty-four years of natural mothering four children and of the experiences of caring for families as a traditional midwife, massage therapist, and herbalist. I am writing, to you, from my heart. The path is never easy, but then again, nothing truly worthwhile is freely given. To surrender your heart and soul to the natural processes of growing, birthing, and nurturing your baby, is a selfless responsibility. You will be rewarded a million times over. Deep mysteries of life and womanhood will be revealed to you. Your life will be blessed with added texture, and a depth of satisfaction will live in you as you watch your baby, and yourself, grow.

You can know that you have loving support for your choices from me, and the other natural mothers of the world. I am honored that you are reading what I have to say. Take what you need from this book as you journey through the process of natural mothering. Blessings!

~Two~

Trusting Intuition

As a natural mother, with your baby being nurtured in your womb, or in your arms, your intuition is one of your greatest friends and will guide you as you make day-to-day decisions regarding the care of motherbaby. You have the ability to access, and trust your intuitive ways of knowing. "The interesting thing is that as soon as you start paying attention to intuition, it does become more available. It's as though it responds to attention, and so it's really not that difficult" (Vaughn, 1998, p.1).

What is Intuition?

So what is intuition? It is a form of intelligence and a fine tuned sense. It is a life force and a way to access our deep inner ways of knowing. Perhaps intuition is a culmination of our entire being. The dictionary defines intuition as, an immediate cognition; sharp insight; the act or faculty of knowing without the use of rational process. "It's a new perception. It's as though it allows us to notice what we haven't noticed and acknowledge what we perhaps already know but have forgotten in some way" (Vaughn, 1998, p.2).

You may experience intuition as a gut feeling, a voice (either your own or another's), a response to move, a peaceful feeling, a flutter or a pain in the heart, while dreaming, an 'aha' experience, or other ways individual to you. How intuition comes to you may be specific for each situation. Some people say that intuition is Divine Spirit (replace this word with God, Allah, Goddess, etc., whatever word works for you) speaking through you.

Ruth Anne defines intuition as *"the language of the heart."* She goes on to explain.

> *I believe the heart is the center of the human body and soul. What I feel in my body is that the heart processes emotions from both internal and external forces. I believe the heart also processes information from the brain. The heart is aware of the external environment such as temperature, safety issues, etc. When as much information as possible is gathered, I believe the heart then sends out an intuitive message. Anyway, this is what my intuition tells me!*

When asked how intuitive knowledge came to them, other natural mothers I interviewed said:

> *I first feel it as a wave: as vibrations running through my body telling me what I am supposed to*

do. It starts out spiritual and then becomes physical. If I am not paying attention, or I do something against what my intuition tells me, I feel it in my tummy. If I don't listen to that I hear voices in my head.

❀

I just feel it in my whole body. I just know what to do.

❀

If fear is involved I feel it in my solar plexus. It says, "Run, you are not safe." If information has been processed and intuition is giving me answers I hear voices in my head. If emotions are being dealt with I feel it in my heart.

❀

An inner drive pushes me forward into behaving in a certain way. Fortunately, this drive, so far, has made right decisions for me. When I first started paying attention to this drive I was worried that it would be wrong. It hasn't been, though, and it has brought me many blessings. I am glad I pay attention to it.

❀

I just feel guided along by something much more than myself. I guess this would be a higher power. It is God telling me what to do.

In our culture, where rational, linear thinking is so prevalent it can be a great change to make decisions based on intuition. How can you make decisions for you and your baby when books, family, friends, the "experts", and mainstream culture all give you information that is counter-intuitive to what your deep ways of knowing tell you? Lorene calls this clouding. She says, *"Clouding means that someone says something against what you innately feel is right. Then you start doubting yourself. You start clouding up. It is important to keep yourself in a place where you don't get clouded. My La Leche League (a national breastfeeding support group) friends didn't cloud me."*

A mother needs support from others for her intuitive ways of knowing. Although intuitive messages may be clear to her, the logistics of how to carry out this intuition may not always be straightforward. Lorene continues, *"Most people who offer advice want to solve a problem the easiest way possible. They want you to feel better as soon as possible. That is not what you want to hear. You want to hear choices for working through a problem until it comes out right. You want to feel encouraged to make the decision that is right for you."*

Paula Reeves writes in her book *Women's Intuition: Unlocking the Wisdom of the Body,*

> It is only when we discover that we are lovely in spite of our 'rebellion' that we can then feel the strength of our uniqueness, our individuality, our selfhood. That being said, it is no easy task for most of us. I have exquisite empathy and respect for the tension contained between the instinctual urge to live life more consciously and the emotional pull to maintain the status quo (Reeves, 1999, p.167).

Following your intuitive voice leads to you being your authentic self, or the person that you truly are. Your authentic self listens to all ways of knowing. However, your linear, rational mind may be threatened by the idea that it may no longer be the supreme decision-maker in your life. It may object to losing control over every situation. You can calm your rational self by assuring your thinking mind that you are not replacing it. Rather, you have found it a new friend, intuition, to work with. That way it won't have to work so hard.

Much information that will be shared with you during your seasons of pregnancy is culturally fear-based. As a whole our society thinks of childbirth as dangerous; an accident waiting to happen. We are asked to believe that we aren't able to give birth without Western medicine there to rescue us. Shelia Kitzinger, a social anthropologist, birth educator, activist and author writes, "We live in a society where it is taken for granted that birth is a medical event which usually takes place in a hospital and is thought about almost exclusively in terms of risk" (Kitzinger, 2000, p.10). While it is true that a small percentage of births do need medical attention, and we all are grateful that medical help is there when needed, most women can give birth naturally with their own strength and wisdom.

Yes, there are risks to giving birth: just as there are risks to living life. There are no guarantees that you will not be injured when you drive in a car or ride a bike. There are no guarantees that you will not choke to death when you eat. And, of course, there are no guarantees that your birth will go exactly as planned. You can base your decisions on every statistic ever published; those numbers certainly don't take individuality into account. Risks don't take into account your individual life story or the experience of the moment.

Using intuition as a knowledge base embraces your life and needs in the moment, and for each life situation. Expanding on your intuition means that you will pay attention to the world and your inner self in a multi-dimensional way. Instead of reacting to fear-based information you surrender to the risks involved in life and focus on how to make the most out of each life experience.

Tribal, or family information, comes from your mother, grandmother, sisters, aunts, family, and friends who often assume that you will follow the ways of the family group. It can be difficult to break away from tribal experiences, especially when past decisions have been made along the dominant cultural paradigm. "Well this is what we did and it always worked for us. Just do what we did!" Tension, misunderstanding, and fear often follow when a woman wishes to follow her own ways of mothering. "*I had to follow the natural mothering path… it was so innate that if I didn't do it I would be going completely against me. There was nothing else in my life that meant anything. I would never be the right person if I did not do this. I would be incomplete. I had to. I just had to. I don't know how to describe how strong this need is for me to follow this path."* These words were spoken from a natural mother who did not have the support of her husband and extended family for her choices.

Many of the mothers I interviewed echoed these sentiments. Alison radically changed her life from being a career woman working in finance after her first baby was born. She says, *" I went from wearing business suits and being in an office every day, to being a full time nursing mother. I had every intention of putting that baby in day-care and going back to work, but I just couldn't leave him!"* Alison has embraced natural mothering so completely that she is often found tandem nursing (nursing a toddler and an infant), nurturing unselfishly, and totally being available for her children.

I am in awe with the strength of these women and their convictions to following a mothering path that was right for them, even if it did cause conflict. Many of these mothers had mentioned that they were willing to live with conflict within their marriage, or without the support of their own parents, if that is what they had to do. Leaving the work place in a time when women are told they "can have it all; marriage, career, home and motherhood" is a courageous act for a woman, especially when that often means that her family will need to be frugal in their spending habits. "Women have been struggling," writes Marianne Williamson in *Enchanted Love*, "to emerge like butterflies from the cocoon into which we were forced for the last few thousand years..."

> ...The journey of our self-actualization—of our rising from the ashes of past physical, mental, and emotional oppression—is clearly one of the major dramas of modern Western civilization. The emergence of true feminine power and glory, while not easy and perhaps rarely accomplished in full, is at least a conscious effort on the part of millions of women (Williamson, 1999, p.89).

I am honored to know women who are so strong within themselves that they do what they need to do to follow their intuitive ways of knowing in spite of conflict. They are paving the way for themselves and for future natural mothers.

Choosing Your Own Path

Each of the mothers I interviewed talked about how they were choosing a path that was quite unlike how they themselves were raised. Many of them had mentioned that they needed to feel as if they were mothering in the way that intuitively seemed right for them, even if this meant straying from how they themselves were raised. Following their intuitive voice kept them happier and more at peace.

They were certain that following this path would be very beneficial for their children. Kim, a mother of five active boys, explained that she hadn't always followed this path to mothering. There was a time when she had put her wants before her children's needs. Kim realized that if she continued to selfishly put her wants first, that would in turn teach her children to be selfish. She turned the situation around when she understood she wanted to exhibit qualities of the nurturing *"God the Father"* to her children and not, *"Me, the selfish parent."* When she learned to listen to her intuitive voice that guided her to natural mothering she not only became less selfish, but also felt *"more at peace with myself."*

It can be difficult to embrace the ideas of natural mothering when your own mother chose a very different way. When the women in your family chose the main stream route, and perhaps had medicated hospital births and bottle-fed babies which they rarely held, it can be confusing and sometimes insulting for them that you would choose a different path. Often people only understand what they themselves have experienced. Or your family may feel as if you don't feel that they did a good job in raising you. Perhaps your own mother has control issues and feels the need to continue controlling your life. Reassure them that you appreciate all of their efforts; past, present, and future. Let them know that there are women following the same path of natural mothering that you are and that you are following your heart.

Lorene talked about how her parents and husband were against her choice of mothering style until they heard a famous author talk about attachment parenting (keeping your baby close to you at all times) on a daytime television show. Attachment parenting is a phrase that is heard now in mainstream media. After watching that television show her family thought it was ok if an "expert" supported the idea. Lorene was hurt that her own family didn't trust her, but would believe an "expert" who in her words, *"Probably never even stayed up all night with a sick baby."* Given time, after family members are able to see that mother and baby are both fine, conflicts may subside. Many mothers stated that they believe their family members and friends even gained a newfound respect for their mothering style.

I understand the pain this can cause as I experienced this first hand when my mother-in-law, a very strong-willed woman, disagreed with my ways of birthing, nurturing, and raising my children. She didn't hold back on saying what she thought either! It was a struggle, and I'm grateful my husband was there to soothe things over. It was my strong trust and belief in my intuitive ways of knowing that kept me steadfast to my mothering style during this difficult time.

Instinct and Intuition

Many people think of instinct and intuition as one and the same. Although intuitive thoughts may transpire from an instinctual response they are not the same. "Intuition is the bridge that connects instinct and all its survival responses with our emotions and their elegant instruction on how to thrive. Intuition is a higher order of embodied response than either instinct or emotion" (Reeves, 1999, p.25). Instincts are consistent within species. Intuition is individual. We all have the same instinct to protect our young, and ourselves, and to react when danger threatens our existence. Instinct causes us to react quickly to the situation. If you perceive a danger to your baby, or yourself, you react. Your heart and breathing rates increase as adrenaline rushes through your body. Every cell in your body says to protect. You experience the fight-or-flight phenomenon.

Ruth Anne tells this story, *When I was pregnant with my first baby, and planning a home birth, my midwives requested that their clients visit their backup doctor for two prenatal check ups. I agreed to this, rationally thinking that it would be a good idea to meet the doctor in case I needed medical attention at some point. When I went to his office my instincts were telling me to leave. I didn't feel safe there. Now logically, I thought that was silly, but my instinctual body didn't think so. My blood pressure was much higher at the doctor's office. I was sweating and my heart was beating fast. I went a few weeks later and the same situation happened. The doctor was concerned about my blood pressure, but I assured him that it was much lower when the midwives took it.*

Why did my body react this way? My belief is that doctors and medicine are for sick people. I wasn't sick, and therefore felt threatened to be in a situation where it felt as if that was the underlying message. I also have such a strong faith and trust in the process of being pregnant, and giving birth at home, that I felt unsafe in an environment that didn't share the same values.

I have seen instinct at work when a woman's labor stops because she doesn't feel safe. Her instincts may be triggered to stall her labor when someone new walks into her birthing nest. Her labor will stop or slow down until she feels safe within her environment again. Or she will not even go into labor until her birthing nest is just the way she needs it.

I once was a midwife for a woman who wouldn't go into labor until her husband returned home from a business trip. Three hours after he walked in the door she began labor and five hours after that they were enjoying a new baby. I've also known women who wouldn't start labor until other visiting family members left. This is instinct. Although it doesn't seem as though any of these situations posed threats, to an instinctual woman, who is near birthing, these situations did make her uneasy. This changes her physiologically, and her birthing energy is shut down until she feels safe again. I have also seen instinct at work when the laboring woman was shown intuitively her baby was not doing well. She felt something was wrong with her baby and stalled her labor.

Types of Intuitive Messages

There are many levels of intuition. In general it is down to earth and used in practical ways every day. However, there are times when deep, intuitive knowledge comes to us revealing magnificent ideas and guides us down a different path than we expected. This happened to me when in my fourth year of music school, and being a new mother, I had a flood of intuition that said, "You must become a midwife!" I felt as if it was shouted from the mountains with great revelry. This was a problem for my rational mind, as I had my life planned out to be a musician. That's all I had ever wanted! I knew not to fight a message that was that strong. I had paid for that mistake in the past, and I had learned my lesson. So here I am today writing this book because I followed my intuition. And yes, I still play music. It was as if a great designer planned my life for me; and I am very happy.

Think of intuition as your guide in everyday decision making. You can learn to check in with yourself, trust your intuition and "voila" the decision is right there for you. This is very handy as a mother because raising children is an ever-changing experience. Just when you think you have a routine down, everything changes. Some days there just isn't time to rationally think about every decision that needs to be made. In many ways it is useless to try to make decisions from your logical brain. You see, your brain spirals into your uterus when pregnant, spirals up to your breasts when breastfeeding, and eventually makes it back up into your head. Trust yourself that your intuition will guide you as you mother your baby.

♥ Think back to a time when you felt as if you had an intuitive experience. What did it feel like? Did the intuition come to you as a voice, an internal vision, or a feeling of peace? What were you doing when the intuition came to you? Did you follow your intuition?

Accessing Intuition

So how can you access and develop your deep ways of knowing?

♥ First of all allow yourself plenty of time to daydream and relax during pregnancy. Quiet your mind. Learn to pay attention to the messages of your inner self. Spend time alone without distractions, out in nature, whenever possible. Sit or lay quietly and just feel your emotions. Where are your different emotions held in your body?

Quiet the body and the mind. Breathe deeply and find the peaceful, quiet place within yourself. Experience the bliss. Strive to maintain this feeling as much as possible throughout your day. Intuitive insights often come during this relaxed state.

♥ Check in with your internal environment. Feel where you are holding any tension. Why is that tension there and what can it teach you? Listen quietly and carefully. Tell the voices of anxiety, doubt, and insecurity to quiet down. Better yet, tell those voices to go take a permanent hike. They do not serve you well. Pay attention to your muscles and where they are holding pain and tension. Are negative emotions finding a home there? Make that home a temporary one by breathing deeply, and then think of relaxing your muscles while whispering for that tension to melt away. We may not have a choice over emotions we feel, but we do have a choice as to how we experience them! Deep ways of knowing will come more easily to you when they are not blocked by physical tension.

Intuition has been called the "sixth sense." During pregnancy all of your senses are magnified. You are an artist creating a new magnificent work of art; your baby. Your heightened awareness of smells, sounds, tastes, touch, sights, and inner knowing serve you well during this time of ultimate creation. Marvel at how deeply your senses can take you. They are there to nourish and protect the motherbaby.

The easiest way to access intuition is to be in touch with your emotions, be relaxed and calm, and to experience your senses. Allow your rational mind to do its work, too. Read and gather information about the childbearing year, but don't allow your rational mind to make all of the decisions. In fact, intuition can be the voice that holistically pieces together all of the information from instinct, emotions, and your rational, logical mind.

Trust the process and know that your deep ways of knowing will serve you well. You will find that when you listen to your inner voice, decisions seem right. Tension that arises when you follow someone else's advice, without truly feeling that that advice is the right choice for you, will dissolve. Heaven is speaking to your soul.

Every day practice relaxation. Check in with your emotions. Discover where your body is holding tension and what the deep inner ways of knowing are telling you. Like all new experiences, listening and following intuition takes practice. Soon you will find that your deep inner ways of knowing come readily to you. Listen to your heart's song by honoring all of the levels of your authentic self. Natural mothering is elemental and brings you to the depths of your intuitive soul.

~Three~

The Seasons of Pregna

Many of life's mysteries are yours to discover during the seasons of your pregnancy. While your baby is growing, nestled in your womb, so too will you grow tremendously in spirit and as a woman. The journey of motherhood has begun the moment you conceive. Consider that this is a life long journey. You are the mother of this new person forever. What a miracle! Of course your intuition will guide you in the protection of this new being. What might you experience while being a vessel for this new person?

THE FIRST SEASON

During the first season, commonly called trimester, you may find that the idea of being pregnant is surreal. It seems as if it isn't possible. It may take many weeks of dreaming about the possibilities before you are able to integrate the reality. This is true whether it is your first baby or your tenth. You may feel a myriad of emotions and it is not uncommon to feel ecstatic one moment and frightened the next. As happy as you may truly be to be pregnant, you may also feel great sadness at the loss of your life as you once knew it. Perhaps you will at you won't be able to take care of a baby. You may have other children and feel as if you won't have enough love and energy to give to a new baby too. Never fear. Your love will not be divided. It will be multiplied!

Life at this time will most likely be very dramatic. Sometimes women go into a state of denial until their deep selves have time to absorb the idea of being a mother. As always, don't be afraid to feel all there is to feel and certainly shed tears of joy and sadness. Accept the fact that your emotions will most likely be spiraling, circling down and up, during the childbearing year. It is also helpful to know that, with time, your emotions will balance themselves.

Physical changes are also profound at the beginning of pregnancy. While your body is adjusting to the hormonal changes needed to keep the process of pregnancy continuing it is very common to feel extremely tired, nauseous, and have tender nipples.

How will you know when your baby will be arriving? You can calculate the general expected time of birth by going backwards three months from the first day of your last menstrual period and adding seven to ten days. For example, if the first day of your last period was May 16, you would go back three months which would be

February. Then add seven to ten days to the 16th of February. This would make the "due date" somewhere around February 23-26. There are several other factors to consider when calculating due dates. One is how long your cycles are, or how many days between periods. Cycles range from 25-32 days. If you have longer cycles it is very possible that your baby will be born later than the calculated due date. Another consideration is family history. Did your mother or sisters have their babies on the early or later side of their due dates? It is well within the normal range for babies to be born two weeks before or after their due date. Be prepared for the latter side of the due date as it seems that most babies are born later on.

Soon after your missed period you will most likely feel tired, sometimes to the point of exhaustion. Take naps during the day whenever possible, and plan to sleep more at night. Extra sleep allows the little placenta to firmly attach to your uterus. Also, while you are sleeping your deep self will have time to process the fact that you are now a mother. So dream of the possibilities that life has to offer you. Revel in your amazing self! In a few weeks the tiredness will lessen.

Remember that all of your senses will be heightened during the seasons of your pregnancy. At the beginning of your pregnancy you may notice that you are particularly sensitive to smell; even smells you ordinarily enjoy. If certain smells make you nauseous try to avoid them. Your body will tell you what to avoid early on. Listen to what it has to say.

Besides your sense of smell telling you what to avoid, your sense of taste also may have a thing or two to tell you. You may feel revulsion to the tastes of certain foods. Avoid them if they make you queasy. Nibble bland, easily digestible foods throughout the day. Many women find that fruits, vegetables, grains and potatoes, are fine for them to eat. I have heard many women say that dairy foods, which create more mucous, make them gag early on in their pregnancy.

During pregnancy your body begins to create more mucous. You will notice more mucous in your nose, vagina, and mouth. This extra mucous is a protective measure and slides harmful microbes right out of your body. Until your body grows accustomed to being pregnant you may want to avoid dairy so that excess mucous doesn't build up and create congestion. Eat green leafy vegetables instead. They have lots of calcium and minerals in them. Remember that these queasy feelings will also soon pass. Hang in there!

Hopefully, queasiness won't turn into vomiting, but if it does there are several natural remedies that may help you out. Sip peppermint or ginger tea. Don't let your stomach get empty. Keep your tea by your bedside and sip it when you wake at night and in the morning before you get out of bed. Some women have said that nibbling on crackers before getting out of bed can also be helpful. I always have on hand a product called Emergence-C. This powder is put into juice or water. The effervescent drink is full of nutrients and is a wonderful up-lifter. You can buy these little packets at health food stores or food co-ops. Look for more remedies in the discomfort chapter.

If you have a strong gag reflex, so strong in fact that you often will vomit, try deep breathing and talking yourself out of it. Perhaps repeat to yourself, "I am fine. I don't need to throw up." Your body may need a bit of reprogramming, but you can remind your gag reflex how to relax.

The good news is that nausea and vomiting of early pregnancy is a healthy sign that the pregnancy is going well. Maybe vomiting is your body's way of eliminating sludge and toxins; both physical and emotional. Brisk walking may help to move the by-products of all of the extra hormones out of your body.

You may not feel like exercising, but try it a few times and see if it doesn't help.

It is not normal, however, to be unable to keep any food or liquids down. If this happens and you begin to feel weak, or are losing weight, talk with your birth attendant. This is a time when further care may be necessary.

During early pregnancy you most likely will experience sore, tender nipples. How exciting it is when you realize that your breasts are much, much more than objects of sexuality. Ruth Anne said, *"I was in awe at the sensitivity of my nipples, and was so proud of my breasts the first time I saw colostrum, the baby's first milk, drip from them during pregnancy."* Yes, breasts are for nurturing. They are life giving, sensual, and sexual.

Usually by the second to third month you will need to urinate more often during the day and at night. This is due to the expanding uterus pressing on your bladder. This is good preparation for being interrupted often. When the baby is in your arms you will need the skill of stopping what you are doing to care for her/him. Don't let frequent urination stop you from drinking lots of water. Remember you are bathing every cell of your body, and your baby's, with water. Plus your baby is floating in amniotic fluid. Keep drinking water!

So much is happening during the first season of pregnancy. The miracle of one egg meeting with one sperm, and in a moment creating the energy and potential of a new human is unimaginable, really. Some women know the moment they conceive. I have heard women say they felt a rush of energy, and a strong intuition, that there was new life. Probably most women don't know that they are pregnant until that first missed period. By then the united cells have rapidly divided as they traveled down the fallopian tube and into the uterus where it is met with the luscious, fertile soil of the endometrium, or lining, of your uterus. The tiny baby is enveloped in a grape-like structure that eventually turns into the placenta, and attaches to the uterus. Here the elixir of life, your blood, will nurture your baby for eight more months.

The uterus starts to move out of the pelvis during the third month and is about the size of a grapefruit. This is the time when you may feel as if you need to urinate more often. As soon as the bulk of the uterus moves out of the pelvis the urge to urinate is often lessened. You also may experience a backache from the expanding uterus. Your baby is now about the size of an apricot.

If your birth attendant owns a doppler, an ultrasound device for listening to baby heart tones, you will be able to hear the heart tones in the latter weeks of the third month. Otherwise you will be able to hear the baby's heart tones at around twenty weeks gestation, or five months with a fetascope. A fetascope is much like a stethoscope, but is designed specifically for listening to babies' heart rates in utero. Some birth attendants also use a pinard horn, which is made from wood or metal and is tube shaped in the middle and bell shaped at each end.

THE SECOND SEASON

By the end of the third month most of the emotional and physical whirlwinds have subsided, or at least greatly lessened. Probably by now you have gotten used to the idea of a new baby coming along. As you move through your days you may awaken out of your deep self and feel more social. You will most likely have more energy and will feel vibrant.

This is a fun time to spend with other mothers following the natural mothering path. You may need to find new friends that you can share your deepest dreams with. Friends can help each other formulate ideas and share in the gathering of information. There is much to learn from one another and the friendship and positive support of other like-minded women is invaluable at this time. The friendship of an older, experienced mother is also wonderful. Her wisdom and stories of natural mothering can teach you the way. Also, observe her style and technique in caring for her baby or children. Does her style resonate with you? Ask your birth attendant if she knows other pregnant women, or new or seasoned mothers that you might be introduced to. Or put up a sign for a natural mothering support group at your food co-op or natural health food store. Attending a La Leche League meeting, a breastfeeding support and information group, is also a way to meet other like minded mothers while you learn the art of breastfeeding, too. La Leche League is a national organization that has groups in many communities. You may have to search around to find the closest group.

You may also find support through *Mothering Magazine*. For over twenty years *Mothering Magazine* has been a valuable resource for natural mothering information. Virtually every article will be of interest to you. This magazine was a great friend to me when I was first pregnant and was instrumental in helping me formulate my ideals of natural mothering. You will find *Mothering Magazine* at many bookstores and newsstands.

If you have access to the internet you will also find informative web sites. Check the resource list for some of my favorites.

Aside from having more energy and feeling more social there are many wonderful physical changes that will happen during the second season of pregnancy. Your uterus will grow out of the pelvis and soon the whole world will notice that you are with child.

You may enjoy the attention bestowed upon you, but beware, many times people you know and even complete strangers feel that it is acceptable to tell you their negative stories. Protect yourself by avoiding these situations, or if you aren't able to avoid these encounters, try this technique. Imagine you and your baby inside a nurturing, protective bubble. Only you can decide what thoughts, emotions, and even people, can enter your bubble. This is your safe haven, your place of refuge. And always remember that someone else's negative story does not need to become your own.

Ruth Anne tells the story of how she was able to negate stories from other women.

Although this may sound arrogant, I would often tell myself that I was stronger, more trusting of the process, and more educated than the woman telling me her nightmare birth story. I remember when I was a few months pregnant with my first baby a woman told me how awful her birth experience was and that I should just plan to go to the hospital early in labor, get an epidural and, in essence, be rescued by the medical staff. It seemed obvious to me that she did not understand or believe in the natural process of labor and birth. I, however, trusted the process fully, and wasn't afraid of pain or feeling strong energy moving through my body. When I told her I was planning a natural home birth she, of course, thought I was crazy.

Be strong in your convictions and don't second-guess your choices. And remember the women throughout the ages who have gone before you. The memory of your ancestors lives in each cell of your body providing you with the knowledge to do this work. In the words of Ralph Waldo Emerson, "What lies behind us and what lies before us are tiny matters compared to what lies within us."

One of the most exciting events of this time is feeling the baby move. What an incredible feeling! Finally the baby seems more real. Now you can integrate the idea that this baby is a living person and not a dream. At first you may notice an internal tickling feeling. It is as if a butterfly is flapping its wings in your uterus. Soon after you will feel little pokes or jabs. This feeling comes from the baby kicking. Also, some babies really like to roll around a lot. Every baby has his/her own energy level, and it is fun to discover the activity level of this special baby that you are growing. You may feel the more active baby at around fifteen weeks and the quieter ones up to the twentieth week.

During the second season of pregnancy the baby is growing at a rapid rate. You most likely will have an increase in your appetite. It is so important that the food you eat has the most nutrition possible so eat a rainbow every day! Nutrition is a key component to a healthy pregnancy. Don't worry about weight gain. If you eat healthy foods when you are hungry you will gain the right amount for you. Most of the mothers I midwife for gain around thirty pounds. Some weeks you may gain more than others may. This is normal. There may be days when you feel as if you just can't eat enough. Soon after you may notice that the baby has a big growth spurt. Listen to your deep body wisdom and you will intuitively know what, and how much, you need to eat.

Pay attention to any food cravings that you have. Why do you think you are craving certain foods? When you crave sugar it may mean that you need more protein. Your body is asking for a quick energy pick up. Or you may crave ice because you need to cool down your internal body heat. You may also desire "comfort" foods, or foods that make you feel better, when stressed. Are there deeper emotional reasons for your food cravings? Perhaps you could discover other ways to comfort yourself.

Stretch marks, the autographs of your pregnancy, often appear on your abdomen and breasts. They are due to the lower layers of skin splitting apart and are a purplish color. The upper layer then stretches giving the skin its shiny appearance. Stretch marks can be itchy so you might want to rub a salve on them. I make a Belly and Butt Balm made from calendula flowers and plantain leaves, infused in olive oil and cocoa butter. This salve is very soothing for stretch marks and itchy skin. After pregnancy it is great for diaper rashes and dry skin.

Your body is changing shape just like an apple growing to protect its seeds—the next generation of the tree. Your cushy abdomen is protecting the seeds of your labor. Your swelling breasts are anticipating the moment when they will take over the nourishment of your baby. You may already be marveling at how your body is swelling. In ancient cultures, fertility figures were often depicted as large, round, full figured women, like the photo on the cover of this book. Roundness and fullness represent nurturing and protection. Yes, your body is changing—that is a fact. You may have to let go of the visual image of the physical person you once were. Now, you are more than that. You are growing, both spiritually and physically, into a mother.

Your sexual desires most likely will greatly change, too. During the first season, fatigue and nausea may have left you feeling as if sex was the last thing on your mind. That may change during the middle months of pregnancy. Many women, but certainly not all, feel a heightened desire for sex now. It's as if your sexual juices are flowing all of the time. Your vagina constantly secretes more mucous and your swollen labia and clitoris are easily aroused. As your uterus expands you may need to explore different positions to find what is comfortable for you. Hands and knees or side lying often work well.

Find other ways of showing affection if you don't feel like having sex. Cuddling and massage are good. Maybe you need more time to warm up to sex. Explain to your partner what your needs are at this time. When you have an orgasm your uterus contracts. This is normal and won't put you into early labor. Perhaps you are afraid that sex will hurt the baby. This is not true. Remember that your baby is well protected and surrounded by amniotic fluid. You may feel that your larger body is not attractive to your partner. This is most likely not true either. A pregnant woman is a beautiful sight to behold!

"During intercourse, childbirth and lactation," writes Michel Odent, in *The Scientification of Love*, "two groups of hormones play a pre-eminent role—the altruistic hormone oxytocin, and the endorphins which can be considered to be our reward system" (Odent, 1999, p. 41). During sexual intercourse oxytocin is what brings us to orgasm. Oxytocin is also the hormone that makes contractions during labor. The euphoric state felt after intercourse is due to endorphins, as is the ecstatic feeling after the birth of your baby. Who knows? Maybe having orgasms during pregnancy is the best childbirth preparation there is! Today, research teams are studying oxytocin receptor sites on uterine muscle. "One can speculate that previous opportunities to release high levels of oxytocin facilitates the development of a greater number of receptors during labour... One can even speculate that self-exploration, flirting and sexual intercourse are ways to prepare the uterine muscle" (Odent, 1999 p.93). So keep those love juices flowing!

During this second season make sure to get plenty of gentle exercise. Listen to your body and don't over do it. Enjoy the fresh air and sunshine while you walk, garden, or swim. Keep stretching, squatting, and moving. Maybe there is a prenatal exercise, yoga, or swimming class in your area. This is a good way to meet other pregnant women, too.

Spend time each day connecting with your baby. Just sit quietly, perhaps in a spot outdoors that feels sacred to you, and feel all there is to feel. Can you believe how much love you feel for this baby? Talk with your baby. Tell the baby your hopes and dreams. Imagine what your baby is doing in your uterus. What position is the baby in? Or, quiet your mind and just be. Intuitions may flow to you.

Sitting in your sacred spot can also be a good place to sort through any ambivalent feelings you may be having. It is not uncommon to have feelings of despair. You may feel anxiety about not being a good mother, or even angry at how your life is changing. Remember that all of your emotions are heightened, so take the good with the bad, the happy with the sad. If negative emotions are deeply troubling you, talk them out with others. This is a time when it is especially important to have the companionship of other mothers.

Although it is easy to get wrapped up in the pregnancy and birth, this second season is a good time to start imagining and thinking about how you are going to care for your baby. Just what does natural mothering mean? Well, you will need to begin to formulate your ideas on holding, feeding, clothing, diapering, sleeping arrangements, health care, etc. Whew! That's a lot to think about.

Let's go through the list. Natural mothers tend to carry, hold, and keep their babies physically close to them at all times. Your baby's senses are nourished and nurtured when being held. Most babies love to be constantly close to you so they can feel your warmth and to continue the rhythm of movement they grew accustomed to in utero. When snuggled on your chest your baby hears the music of your heartbeat and smells your sweet breast milk.

Breast milk is, of course, the milk nature intended for the human baby. Although breastfeeding is natural, it is also learned by watching other women nurse their babies. If you didn't grow up around nursing mothers I strongly suggest you find a La Leche League group to visit while pregnant. There you will learn a lot about the art of breastfeeding just by observing.

Gathering baby clothes and supplies is fun. Can you believe your little person will wear those tiny newborn clothes? Dress your baby in soft cotton clothes. Organic cotton baby clothes are now available in many stores. Many people like to give the baby a gift, so start a wish list now and let family and friends know what your preferences are.

What kind of diapers will you use? There are many arguments for and against both cloth diapering and disposable diapers. Of course there are environmental issues to consider. It takes approximately six to seven trees to make enough disposable diapers for a baby for approximately two years and thousands of gallons of water are used to wash cloth diapers. Environmentally speaking, you have to choose which resources you wish to use more of when considering diapering.

Sometimes the comfort of the baby gets overlooked in the decision making process. Marisol says, *"When I started using cloth sanitary napkins, instead of disposable ones, I realized how much more comfortable the cloth napkins are. I believe babies would prefer the feeling of cloth on their bottoms way more than scratchy disposable diapers, too. Although the initial cost of cloth diapers and sanitary napkins is more, in the end cloth costs considerably less."*

Also, consider that a diaper is an article of clothing. Typically a cloth-diapered baby gets changed more often, as fluid stays next to the skin. With disposable diapers there is a temptation to change the baby less often because fluid is absorbed into the lower layers of the diaper.

Many natural mothers prefer to sleep right next to the baby in the family bed. Some people are very opposed to babies sleeping in the same bed as their mothers, so be ready to hear some opposition. There is a good bit of fear that the baby could be smothered by bedding or rolled onto and suffocated. In the same way that you are aware of the edge of the bed and don't roll off at night, so too will you be aware of where your baby lies.

Also, people are afraid that a baby will be spoiled with too much attention. It seems natural that a baby would feel more secure and sleep better if she/he were near warmth and could sense her/his mother nearby. This is not true for all babies though. Sometimes babies prefer to sleep by themselves. As always, listen to what your baby has to say. Yes, babies have their own opinions. I have heard mothers say they also sleep better when the baby is next to them because they can hear the baby breathing and know that all is well. Other mothers have said that both they and their baby sleep better if the baby sleeps in a bassinet. Keep your options open and know that the right way is what is right for your baby, you, and the entire family.

I have seen many arrangements of beds for family sleeping. A king size bed is wonderful, but if you don't have one, pushing mattresses together also works well. Futons or mattresses can also be set right on the floor. You could also purchase a bed extender. This is a tiny mattress with a frame that slides between the box spring and regular mattress of your bed. There are safety bars along the three sides. This allows the baby to sleep nearby while also having her/his own space. Another added benefit to the family bed, or sleeping nearby to one another, is that it is easier to nurse in the early months when the baby is nearby. When the baby is hungry you can simply roll on your side and doze as the baby nurses.

It is necessary to also begin thinking about health care for your baby. Have you developed your own philosophy of natural health care? (Later chapters in this book can assist you in organizing and developing your beliefs surrounding health care.) What healing modalities are you most attracted to? Will you use herbs, massage, homeopathy, chiropractic, when the baby is not feeling well? Do you truly believe that most illnesses will take care of themselves? Will you support the body during its healing process? It can be hard to be level headed when your baby is sick. You may feel that you won't be able to handle caring for a sick baby, especially the first few times. In many communities there are natural health care providers who can help you during times of illness. It is best to search them out now, before you need them.

This is also a good time to think about vaccinations. (More on vaccinations is covered in the Motherbaby Moon Time chapter.) Research the topic so that you can make your own informed decisions regarding whether or not to vaccinate.

Many medical doctors are learning to approach health care more holistically. Try to find one in your area that you can consult with if needed. You may want to purchase some resource books on natural healing. Check the resource list at the end of this book.

Have you thought about people you wish to have with you as labor companions? Labor and birth is a sensual and sexual time. Most often women prefer as few people as possible. If you choose to have other people attend besides your partner and midwives it is very important that they are supportive of your choice of birthplace and your desire for natural childbirth. Labor progress can be impeded if you are not entirely comfortable with the people that are in the environment. You may realize once you begin labor that you don't want other people there, even though you have invited them. Keep your options open by explaining to friends and family that you may or may not call them depending upon how you feel at the time. They may be disappointed, but will understand.

THE THIRD SEASON

The last three months of your pregnancy are a time of great anticipation. You will go deep into your inner self as you prepare for labor. It is normal to not feel very social. You are concentrating on the fact that you are about to give birth. Give yourself all of the time alone you need and work out any issues, if possible, you may have before labor. Childhood and relationship issues sometimes emerge. If you aren't able to talk through problems with a person close to you, write about these issues. Often writing can help to clarify problems. Remember all of your relationships are changing as you become a new mother.

Also, now is the time to work through deep fears that you may have surrounding the birth. It is normal to feel fleeting moments of fear. What I am talking about here are the deep-rooted fears that paralyze you when you think about them. Remember that fear sets our instincts into motion. The fight-or-flight response can be activated and has the potential to shut down the labor process. Fear must be replaced with trust. Now that certainly is easier said than done.

Try out this method and see if it works for you.

♥ First you must clearly identify what your fear is. It may be fear of moving through the process of birth. Perhaps you can't imagine pushing or your perineum stretching. Are you afraid that you or your baby will die during labor and birth? Do you feel that your body isn't capable of birthing? Are you afraid of the intensity of labor? Do you feel that you won't be able to be a good mother?

♥ Write down your fear. Now ask yourself, "Why am I afraid of this?" List all of the reasons you are afraid. Now use your rational mind to think of reasons why your fear is unwarranted. For instance, if your deep fear is that you won't be able to handle the enormous energy of labor write, "I am afraid of contractions and the intensity of labor." Now list your reasons why you are afraid. "I don't handle pain well. I have a low threshold for pain. Other women tell me that labor is unbearable. I don't know what it will feel like, etc."

♥ Now use your rational mind to gather information. List this information. "If I stay relaxed my body will release endorphins, natural morphine, that will bring me to an altered state and lessen my perceptions of the sensations that I will be feeling. Throughout time women have birthed naturally and they have been fine. Massage, being in water, breathing, and the freedom to be in different positions will assist me in moving through the intensities of labor. Nature never will give me more than I can handle, etc."

♥ Now make a list of positive statements you can recite over and over to yourself. "I am strong. My body was made to birth this baby. I have inherited the strength from time eternal of all of the women who have birthed before me. I have done the best I could to prepare myself. Labor is hard work and I am not afraid of hard work." Repeat these positive statements over and over to yourself. When fear rears its fierce head at the door, calm it by reciting these words to yourself. It may take days, but soon fear melts away and is replaced with trust and a strong belief that you can do this. Fear will not hold you back from having the birth experience that you desire.

During the seventh month you usually are still moving well and will feel good. As the baby grows and puts pressure on your stomach you may experience heartburn. You also may start noticing that it is harder to breathe and you have shortness of breath due to pressure on the lungs. The baby is moving a lot; there is still room to roll from side to side. Your baby is two to three pounds and twelve to fourteen inches long.

As the baby grows longer and gains weight, you may begin to feel uncomfortable. During the eighth month it can be harder to find comfortable positions for sleeping. Try having lots of pillows to support your belly, and put a pillow between your knees so that there will be less strain on your lower back. Make sure when you sit up that you lie on your side and push up with your elbow. Using your elbow to push yourself up lessens stress on your abdominal muscles. It begins to be rather cumbersome to move, but keep moving! Keep up with your gentle exercise and stretching. You need to stay physically strong.

You may notice that your joints are beginning to feel looser. This is due to a hormone called relaxin, which does exactly what its name says; it relaxes your joints and tissues. The release of relaxin is a great thing. During labor it allows the pelvic bones to open up to allow more room for the baby to pass through. It most likely will feel odd to you while pregnant though to have joints that feel like jelly!

You might experience leg cramps especially in your calves. This can sometimes be intense. If you get a cramp, gently stretch your toes upward toward your head. This will stretch the muscles. Leg cramps can be due to a lack of available calcium. You can easily add more greens to your diet to increase your calcium.

Your baby will reach a weight of around four to seven pounds and gain several inches in length during the eighth month. A baby has less room to roll around now and will most often settle into a head down position. Really pay attention to the position of your baby. If you take time each day to deeply focus on your baby, your intuition will tell you what position your baby has chosen.

During the ninth month you may feel ripe and you may feel ready to no longer be pregnant. As it becomes cumbersome to move, you may long to have your body back. There isn't much room for the baby to move now and this is why your baby will probably find one position and will just stretch when needed. It's no wonder that it is harder for you to move now. Your baby has grown from two little cells into a little person weighing several pounds. Your baby is growing a special kind of fat called brown fat. This fat is an energy reserve and is metabolized after birth until your milk comes in. Your baby has also grown eighteen to twenty-one inches long.

Lightening, which is the process of the baby moving deeper into your pelvis, will give more room for your stomach and less room for your bladder. So you may be able to eat more at each meal, but you will also need to urinate more often. Lightening usually occurs a few weeks before birth with your first baby and may not happen until labor with subsequent babies. You may develop quite a waddle as the baby's head moves deeper into your pelvis. The pressure of the baby's head on the cervix helps to soften it and assists in opening up your pelvis. Warm-up contractions, commonly called Braxton-Hicks contractions, may be a common occurrence in the last month. These warm-up contractions, at first, may be felt as tightness in one area of your uterus. As time goes on the muscle fibers become more co-ordinated, and you will feel the entire uterus contract. If you have already given birth you can expect to experience warm-up contractions often during this month.

The round ligaments that attach to the top of your uterus on both sides, and attach again at your pubic bone, sometimes stretch and send out a fleeting, sharp shooting pain. This may happen if you twist your body or move quickly. Round ligaments are much like the ropes that hold down an inflated hot air balloon. They anchor the uterus and keep it from tipping.

As the days go on it is not uncommon to experience various aches and pains. You may have sharp shooting pains in your vagina and tension in your muscles. A small muscle in the hip called the piriformis may pinch the sciatic nerve. When this nerve is squeezed, pain is sent down the leg. Numbness down the leg can also occur. Sitting on a tennis ball can help relieve discomfort. Find the tender, sore spot; usually this spot is in the middle of your buttocks. Position the ball on the sore spot and then sit on it. This is a "hurts so good" sort of feeling. The sensation you feel may at first be intense. Persevere and sit on the ball for a few minutes. Relief should come soon. You can use the ball anywhere on the body where there is muscle tension.

See if you can find a massage therapist who owns a pregnancy massage table. This table has a hole in the upper third of it. A harness fits in the hole to support your belly. If your therapist doesn't have a pregnancy table she/he will have you lie on your side supported with lots of pillows. Pay attention to where you are holding muscle tension. Are your shoulders and neck relaxed?

Well into the third season of your pregnancy you will undoubtedly be preparing your nest. As the days move closer to the blessed event you will go deeper into yourself. You will prepare your nest, your birthing room, the way you intuitively need it. It is important to feel totally safe and comfortable in your home. If you will be birthing in a birth center or hospital you might want to bring your own music and machine to play it on, and anything else that will help you feel comfortable. Some women bring their favorite essential oils, battery operated soft lights, flowers, pictures, sheets, etc.

You will definitely develop your patience during the last days of pregnancy. Waiting for this new person to be in your arms can seem like an eternity. Learning patience will definitely serve you well. Patience is a hallmark of mothering. You may be tired of being pregnant, but just remember, no one stays pregnant forever!

The fruit of your seed is now ripe and ready to leave the vine. You are ready to begin the journey of labor and birth. You will pass through another dimension where there are mysteries and miracles that you will understand as you come through the other side. Blessings on your journey!

~Four~

The Journey of Birth

As the journey of birth draws near you will find that you go deeper and deeper inside yourself. It is of utmost importance that your rational, thinking mind is quieted as your intuitive and instinctual selves take over. Thinking can actually slow the birth process because it hinders the release of oxytocin. Remember that the process of giving birth is in some ways very similar to the process of sexual arousal and orgasm. Does the sexual process work well if you are thinking about other things? Of course it doesn't. You have to let your mind go, and just feel and be. During sex you feel energy rising and passion pulsing to the deepness of your being. The whole process is instinctual and intuitive. Your thinking, rational brain shuts off. It needs to be the same while birthing.

The process of giving birth is elemental and takes you to the depths of your soul. Not only is a baby born, but also a new woman, and a new family is born. You are giving birth to yourself as a new mother. Yes, giving birth is an awesome task, but one that you must believe your body and soul is capable of doing. Just remember that you will never be given more than you can handle. You will be amazed at the inner strength you have. You are an amazing miracle of womanpower!

Strive to maintain a deep inner peace during the days leading up to your birth. Feeling peaceful allows the inner circuits of energy to flow smoothly through your body and creates the perfect environmental physiology for your labor hormones as they increase. Being a peaceful, open vessel really allows for birthing energy to open up and flow!

Quiet any feelings of worry, anxiety, fear, or even over-excitement. Check in with your intuitive self to understand why you are feeling these feelings. Do you truly know that everything is fine or are you worried that something is not right? If everything is fine, replace those feelings with trust. Find positive words that you can repeat to yourself over and over. For instance, if you feel anxiety over the stretching of your perineum you could tell yourself that "my bottom is made to stretch around my baby". Keep telling yourself that. Soon you will believe it. I can't stress enough how important it is to replace fear with trust.

The process of pregnancy and birth is amazing and almost always works just fine. However, if you are experiencing intuitive messages that tell you everything is not fine, listen to that message. Talk with your birth attendant and tell her your concerns. Get further medical checks if need be. The idea is that you enter into labor calm and serene.

It is also important to be well rested in the days leading up to labor. Certainly you are getting up at night to urinate often. Sometimes it is hard to go back to sleep. If that is the case, make sure that you are able to take naps during the day. Schedules, or lack there of, will take on a new meaning when the baby is born. Sleeping during the day and night prepares you for the new rhythm of life you will experience. Remember that new babies don't know the difference between night and day. During the first few days you and your baby may sleep as much during the day as at night.

Giving love, and feeling loved, are also very important to the process of preparing for labor. Oxytocin is secreted any time you feel loved. It is released when you feel deep love for your partner, other children, and all life in general.

As the labor draws near many women find that they don't feel very social. When you are with others it is especially important to surround yourself with people who are supportive of your birth environment and desire for natural childbirth. Just as in pregnancy you don't need to hear, or feel, fear and negativity surrounding labor and birth from others. Fear will increase adrenaline, which may slow or stop the flow of oxytocin. You certainly don't want your "love hormones" to stop flowing.

Many women find that they have an instinctual urge to prepare their "birthing nest" in the days leading up to labor. You may have a burst of energy and want to clean your house or tidy up. Or you may feel the need to finish up any projects. If everything is in order you may want to begin a creative project such as writing, drawing, sewing, etc. While in the process of creating you tap into your intuitive mind as you are drawn into yourself. Perhaps you could write your thoughts and feelings about being pregnant or make your baby a little quilt.

For the past few days, or weeks, you probably have been experiencing warm-up contractions, commonly called Braxton-Hicks contractions. You may feel a tightening of the uterus for several seconds, then a relaxation, and then feel the same tightening a few minutes later. Sometimes the uterus contracts in one area and not others. Eventually you will notice that the entire uterus is tightening. It is common to experience warm-ups in the evening. These contractions are coordinating each of the muscle fibers to work together. I like to call them warm-up contractions because they do just that; they prepare, or warm-up, your uterus for the strong work ahead, and also assist your spirit/body/mind to integrate and prepare for labor. Soon warm-ups start to come at other times during the day and night, may last longer, and be closer together. You may experience these warm-ups for an hour or as long as several hours at a time.

It is easy to get excited while wondering if this is the beginning of real labor. One way to tell if you are in true labor is to change positions. During warm-up labor the contractions will stop when you change position. True labor contractions will often get stronger with a change of position.

The mucous plug may come out several days or hours before you begin labor. The mucous plug comes from the neck of the cervix and seals off your uterus. You may find that the piece of mucous is several inches long, or it may come out in smaller pieces. When it is blood tinged it is called the "bloody show." The blood comes from capillaries that have broken open as your cervix effaces, or shortens, and begins to dilate, or open up. This is normal and is a good sign that labor energy is building.

Let's look at other differences between warm up labor and true labor.

Warm Up Labor

1. Gentle contractions that don't intensify in strength.
2. Contractions stop with mother's change of position.
3. Contractions don't get closer together.
4. Mucous plug may come out and may be pink or brown tinged.

True Labor

1. Contractions intensify in strength.
2. Contractions most likely will get stronger with a change of position.
3. Contractions get closer together.
4. Mucous plug may come out and be pink tinged or have red blood mixed with it.
5. You may have diarrhea.

The natural process of giving birth is unique to each individual. Remember that labor and birth are elemental. You are the vessel for giving life, and nature has her own ideas of when your baby should be born. I'm sure there are many factors involved in the process that we aren't even aware of. Could it be that the heavens open up to bring you birthing energy when the moon is full? Or in the divine plan does your baby need to be born at a certain time? Who knows? Just as a seed sprouts when the earth is warm enough, and there is water to swell the outer shell, so too will your body, and your baby's body, wait for the "ripe" moment.

Often mothers prefer to be alone or to have quiet attendance of their partner and/or midwife. Lorelei tells the story of how she felt about others being with her while in labor.

> *I mostly needed to be by myself in labor. It seemed like I was guided along. Is that intuition? I don't know, but it moved me through labor. I knew when it was time to do things. When my first baby was born I had just moved to this area, and I didn't have anything, or anyone, close to me. Everything was new in my environment. My husband and two midwives were with me. My husband slept through most of the labor. I don't even know if my midwives knew that they were a calming presence for me. They just supported me and reassured me that everything was fine. The second birth I didn't want anybody familiar around me. I didn't want other people's emotion*

there. I didn't want to be the center of attention of other people. I just needed to do my work by myself.

As your birthing energy builds you may feel as though there is just you and the eternal mother, and that you, and she together, will go through the journey of birth. Ruth Anne tells the story of her birth experience.

While in labor it seemed as though I was floating above my body. I could sense or feel other women with me, but they weren't in the room. I saw in my mind's eye women of long ago birthing with me, but they weren't actually having babies. They were simply feeling it with me and were there with me. It was as if they were my birthing angels.

Please wait patiently as your birthing energy is growing and ripening. Time is not a concern for you as you flow through warm-up labor. Continue on your days just living life. Make sure you are well nourished and rested. Take walks and enjoy nature, work on a project, clean your house, read, etc.

Accept each warm-up contraction and know that these contractions have a useful purpose because they are effacing your cervix. The cervix is normally around three to four centimeters long. During effacement the cervix gradually gets shorter until it is very thin. It can take several hours to days for your cervix to efface. Usually, if you are having your first baby, it takes days.

Nature gives a first time mom lots of time to get used to warm-up contractions. When your birthing energy increases your cervix will begin to dilate. Cervical dilation means that the opening of your cervix goes from a fingertip opening to ten centimeters open.

If you have any deep concerns or fears you may be processing through them at this time. Tears often surface. Let those tears flow as they wash away your emotions. Often after a good cry a peaceful calm surrounds you. Breath deeply with that feeling as peacefulness embraces you. Quiet your mind from endless chatter. Let yourself feel as though you were liquid.

I have always thought of labor as a gradual strengthening of birthing energy. To me it is a mistake to compartmentalize the process into stages. You may have heard about 1st stage (labor), 2nd stage (pushing and birth), and 3rd stage (birth of placenta). First stage is further divided into three stages: early, active, and transition. A natural mother, one who goes with the flow of life, understands that there are no divisions of the rhythms of labor and birth. The process almost always begins gradually and builds into a sensual, climatic finale.

As your birthing energy builds, the warm-up contractions become more regular. Keep on moving and participating in the flow of life. This will take as long as it takes. Understandably, if you are a first time mom you may begin to feel anxious while experiencing the process moving forward.

Sometimes women say that the beginning of regular contractions is the hardest part of labor. You may hope that this is as strong as labor gets, and can't imagine that contractions can become any stronger. Know that if you are talking in-between contractions it will be a while before your baby is born. Stay in the moment, and welcome each contraction one at a time. When contractions become more intense you may need to experience a few before you settle into them.

You'll soon find coping techniques that work for you. Here are some that have assisted other mothers.

♥ Imagine that you are swimming in the ocean. Each wave is a contraction. You ride on top of each wave as the energy moves towards you, through you, and past you. If you get caught off guard, and a wave sneaks up on you, you may feel consumed and swallowed by the great force. This is a time to breath deeply and work to get back on top of the wave of contractions. Just as you would allow the wave to carry you through so too will your uterus carry you. The rest of your body is there for the ride.

♥ Sometimes women like to sway or rock their hips while standing or being on hands and knees.

♥ Water is very calming and relaxing for some women. Standing in the shower or sitting in a tub of body temperature water might be what helps you through labor.

♥ Chanting through labor can be helpful.

♥ Massage of your back or feet can be very relaxing.

♥ Be sure your environment is peaceful. Dim lights and a warm room can assist in keeping you in your deep inner self.

♥ Breath deeply.

♥ Keep your eyes open.

♥ Encouraging words from others are invaluable.

What does labor feel like? It is a gradually intensifying elemental force moving through you. It feels as though your body is a thunderstorm, or giant waves. The rhythmic contractions you feel are a great force moving through you. Just as in a thunderstorm, your energy builds, and pulses, and pressure expands. You enter further into the universe as the universe enters further into you. This journey is intense and hard work. If you believe that you will be all right, and that you can ride out the weather, your journey will be much more bearable.

Often when I am attending a birth I can see white light stream from above a woman and enter her through the very top of her head. The intensity of light builds as the laboring mother's contractions increase in strength. Sometimes I wonder if it is this light energy that creates contractions. Whatever the purpose of this light it is apparent that there are mysteries and greater forces of nature moving through the birth process.

The following poem honors the connection of a laboring woman and nature.

The Weathered Mother

I stand alone, naked before the spring storm.
It is quiet— I listen with open ears,
to the swelling silence.
All life is open to anticipation,
And wondering of what is to come.

Pressure builds—the wind gathers its momentum.
It blows and twists and pushes at me.
I want to run and hide,
But there is no shelter.

I only have my body, myself,
To weather the storm.
Fear overcomes me,
As mounting tension rises.

The dark clouds roll in.
They are angry. They are powerful.
They push all that is before them,
Out of the way.

The rain begins to pelt on me.
There is no place to hide.
I stand here raw,
Just me, myself, on my own.

I stand alone, naked at the shore of the ocean.
Drawn into the sea,
I am engulfed in the mounting waves,
Sucked under by the pull of the undertow.

I learn to no longer walk into the force
But instead, I ride on the rhythm of the waves.
Surfacing, and calmly,
Riding out the wave energy.

Panic rises in my soul,
As the force of the waves rise.
I have lost my way.
I am being sucked in. I might drown.

But I do surface; I do survive.
I vow to pay more attention,
To the rising waves.
But no, oh no; divine spirit, help me.

This tension is more than I can bear.
I struggle to find the eye of the hurricane,
Where it is peaceful,
Where I can ride out the storm.

I stand alone, naked in the parched desert.
Elements in the raw, fire without a flame.
Moves me forward,
To escape the heat.

In the far distance I see,
At the foot of a mountain,
The shade of pine trees.
Calling me to move forward.

I strive to keep moving,
And trust that my parched body,
Has the strength to push ahead,
To reach my destination.

Somehow I must find the strength
To carry on,
The pulse of my soul, and blood and guts,
Keeps me moving.

I stand naked in the pristine snow.
Having reached the end of my seasonal journey,
I marvel at the holiness,
And purity of the new fallen snow.

©Janice Marsh-Prelesnik, 2004

Pain is the name our culture so unwisely gives to this elemental energy moving through a laboring woman. While I don't deny that the physical sensations of labor are strong and intense, I do believe that we are better served by using a word other than pain to describe what labor feels like. Or at the very least, we can recognize that there are different kinds of pain. In the book *Sacred Cycles; The Spiral of Women's Well-Being*, Sara Wickham writes,

> Perhaps we become confused by the fact that there is more than one kind of pain; the kind of pain that tells us that something is not right with our body, and the kind of pain that comes from doing hard work for a long time. We "know" that birth is painful because we grow up with this belief so entrenched around us that we cannot possibly help learning this. How different would it be to grow up in a village where the women experienced joy during their births? (Wickham, 2004, p.89).

We must learn to differentiate body sensations. There are different kinds of pain. In everyday life, pain is a messenger that tells us to pay attention to our bodies. Pain can be caused by a myriad of reasons and is useful for encouraging us in bringing our bodies back to balance.

Many people consider any pain bad and choose to try to eliminate it as quickly as possible. "There is little doubt we have reached a point in our social and cultural development where we have a tendency to medicate lots of aspects of our lives. There are drugs or treatments available for almost everything that should be removed from our lives" (Wickham, 2004, p.89).

If you consider that the sensations or pain in labor are those of hard work, and not the kind of pain that signals something is wrong, you will be well on your way to working through labor. My Grandma Sayer, a hard working farmwoman, always told me that giving birth was like a day off from her regular hard physical labor work on the farm. She claimed that birthing was easier and that she loved being taken care of for a few days.

Lorna Davies, a midwife, mother, and marathon runner, compares labor and birth to running a marathon. Lorna writes,

> The role of the supporter would appear to me to be of equal importance in each event. The focus on the encouragement of those around you becomes increasingly significant as the toil continues, and the complete trust and belief in that support is invaluable.... The point at which the support of

the crowd became so significant can be compared to transition [near the end] in labor.

Lorna goes on to say, "The nutritional requirements for marathon running and laboring women is an interesting association..." She wrote that a high calorie, isotonic drink, is imperative and because of liquid nutrition she was able to complete both processes. "Crossing the finishing line and pushing my babies out also brings to mind a range of parallel encounters. The tears, the triumph, the sense of relief, the exhaustion, the pain! I was able to share this glory with partner and friends after my babies had been born" (Davies, 2001, p.1-3).

While in labor you may feel a sharp sensation in your lower back and hips. Sometimes this sensation radiates down the legs. Massage may help the pain. Getting in a tub of water or a birthing pool will likely lessen the sensation too.

As the baby moves down you will feel intense pressure in your pelvis. When your perineum (between your vaginal opening and anus) stretches you will feel a burning sensation. This feeling is similar to opening your mouth wide and then stretching your lips with your fingers.

As you surrender to the forces of labor you will discover that the creative energy of labor and birth is the essence of the embodied female and reveals many mysteries of life. Open yourself and surrender to the immense energy. You must remember that you will be cared for by Divine Spirit and others who are with you as the forces flow through you.

The great news is that as you release more oxytocin, the love hormone, you also will release more endorphins, or natural morphine. You see, nature provides for you. As your birthing energy flows stronger your coping partner, endorphins, are with you and provide you with the feeling of being calm and far away. Endorphins allow you to feel as if you are in a dream world where the intensity of the experience becomes much more manageable. If your labor progresses naturally, without interference and intervention, your body will provide endorphins.

Fear and interference in the process brings on adrenaline, which alters the physiological processes of labor. When adrenaline is released the body is sent a message that all is not safe. Your body will go into a protection mode with a desire to stop labor until all is well. This is very confusing for the body and leads to internal struggles.

As the nature of contractions build momentum, and your endorphins are released, you may feel as if you are floating through labor. Some mothers talk about having an out-of-body experience. This feeling comes from endorphins and really carries you through the hard work of labor. As your birthing energy grows to its final destination of birthing your senses are heightened more than any time in your life.

Don't be surprised if you like to be touched one minute and not the next. Or you may feel cold one second and then hot the next. You may be astonished to discover that your normally modest self doesn't care a bit if you are naked while giving birth. You never know what paths the journey of labor will take you on! Just believe that you will reach your destination. Trust this amazing process. And remember, no one stays pregnant and in labor forever! You too will come through to the other side.

As your birthing energy climaxes you must surrender to the powers moving through you. You can't control it or deny it. It is natural to feel, and even voice, "I can't do it." Energy mounts as your cervix opens the last bit and birthing energy crashes and spirals down through you. It is as if you are caught in a twenty-foot wave with the enormous force pushing and pulling, sucking, and slapping at you. Perhaps you will be sputtering a bit, but that's okay. Surrender to the intensity of late labor. Breathe deeply through the contractions and know that you can do it. Take the time to rest in-between contractions and gather your strength for the next.

When your cervix completely opens up, the nature of the birthing energy changes. You will feel more awake; more bright eyed and alert. Continue to breathe as the baby begins to move down through your vagina. Pay close attention to what your body tells you to do and which position your body wants to be in. You will feel an increased pressure as the baby's head pushes on your rectum. You may not feel an overwhelming urge to voluntarily push. That's fine. Just let your uterus move the baby down. Many women just breathe their babies out. However, you may need to push quite hard, especially for your first baby.

There is no right technique or position for pushing. Squatting, side lying, standing, hanging squat (the mother stands and is supported facing away from another who is holding her under her arms), semi-sitting, hands and knees, are all positions that you may wish to try. Your body will tell you intuitively which position is best for the moment. If and when your body has an overwhelming urge to push, follow the leads, and bear down.

It is exciting when the baby's head begins to appear. Often, especially with a first baby, a bit of the head will show only to slide back up in-between contractions. This can be discouraging when you feel as if the baby is going backwards! This is normal and allows time for the baby to have a nice head massage while your vagina stretches. Soon enough the presenting part of the head, which is usually the upper back part of the head, emerges and begins to stay out in-between contractions. You will feel an intense burning feeling on your perineum (the area between your vaginal opening and anus). You may like some warm olive oil on your bottom at this time. This oil may not help prevent tears, but most women love how soothing it feels.

As the baby's head begins to emerge try to not force the head out with strong pushes. You may need to blow out with contractions. This gives your bottom time to stretch and moves mucous out of the baby's nose and throat. Just when you feel as if you can't possibly stretch any more the baby will lift her/his face up and the whole head will be born. Wow, what a relief! The climax is over and you can have a breather for a moment. Time can seem like an eternity between the birth of the head and the rest of the baby. The rest of the baby may follow quickly, or it may take a couple of minutes before the next contraction comes.

The shoulders and body usually birth quickly with the next contraction. Suddenly, you are experiencing the magical moment of having your baby in your arms. The moment you first meet your baby is an amazing time. You and your baby are fully alert as adrenaline rushes through both of your bodies. Such a flood of emotions will wash over you. It is amazing how the umbilical cord is just long enough for the baby to be up in your arms.

The immensity of emotions you will feel really are indescribable. Elation, joy, ecstasy, and immense love are some words that come to mind. You will remember this moment the rest of your life. Curiosity to know this new person will flood your entire being. What kind of environment do you wish for your baby's first impressions of life on earth? Soft lighting, a very warm room, and quiet voices are important for you and the baby to gently adjust.

Babies are born with a rather mottled look to their skin. As your baby begins to breathe, she/he will gradually begin to pink up from the chest radiating outward. With delayed cord cutting your baby will still be receiving oxygen from the umbilical cord for a minute or two. This is nature's way of providing a gradual transition for the baby.

Babies are very curious and will open her/his eyes and look right at you. Babies often make little cooing sounds and sometimes cry. The intelligence and wisdom of a baby just a few minutes old is profound.

In the next few minutes you will feel some cramping contractions. Pay attention to these as the placenta, the internal grandmother, is beginning to separate. Give some gentle pushes when you feel these contractions. It usually takes about twenty minutes for the placenta to fully separate and be born. Birthing the placenta is not intense like birthing the baby. Pay attention to body signals at this time. Honor and respect the placenta and keep in mind that this is an important time for your safety.

Once the placenta is born you can snuggle up with your baby undisturbed. Sometimes babies like to nurse right away. Other times they just like to nestle and nuzzle right next to the breast. Keeping the baby right with you continues the process of the release of oxytocin. This initiates the release of the placenta and keeps the uterus contracted so that you won't bleed too much. Your baby will most likely be very alert for an hour or two. It is important to have uninterrupted bonding time and to integrate the depth of the experience you have just gone through. Soon you will both be ready for a blissful sleep. You both came through the journey and out the other side. Shout it from the mountains. This is a great day; the birthday of your baby and the birthday of you as a new mother. Congratulations!

~Five~

The Season of Motherbaby Moon Time

Oh, sweet bliss; that magical time when you first greet the flesh of your flesh and the bones of your bones. Savor the moment, as it will forever be etched in your entire being.

❂

Relish the fresh smell of your baby, the feel of soft newborn skin, the radiance of the first breaths, the essence of this unique human being. For me, as a midwife and a mother, this moment in time is the most glorious of all human experience. During these first few minutes, when motherbaby, and the entire family, fall deeply in love, a healthy foundation for a lifetime of human experience is formed. No moment in time is more important for the future of human life on the planet!

This bonding time makes way for an easier transition into motherbaby moon time. During this season, or the first few weeks after birth, it is important that a safe space is created for the new family to get to know one another. It is best if this space can remain much the same as the birthing environment that you created: peaceful, very warm, softly lit, and filled with harmonious, soft music. It is important to gently ease the newborn into living in this world. This is a sacred, holy time. Creating this sacred space is an important job for the husband, partner or any other person who is close to motherbaby. The job of this person is to protect the space for the motherbaby unit. Never underestimate the importance of having a person providing and protecting at this time as the unity of the motherbaby depends on this person.

During this transition time when your body is healing, and you begin to make milk, you also will be dealing with tremendously deep emotions. Your intuitive self takes over as you spend time learning how to care for the uniqueness of this new baby. For a smooth transition the motherbaby needs protection from over stimulation, outside microbes, and general chaos from the outside world. The two of you, as one, need time to explore one another and dance with the rhythms of your special relationship.

Providing this safe space may mean that outside help, perhaps from family or friends, is needed. Being mothered yourself, so that you can mother your baby is so important. For at least a week after the birth you should try to do nothing else but care for your baby and yourself. That is all. Allow other people to bring you food and drink. It is best if all household chores, including cleaning, cooking, and laundry are done by someone else. Also, have a plan for childcare for other children. I have heard many fathers and partners comment that they became closer to their older children after the birth of a new baby.

Perhaps a community of friends or family could organize care and provide meals and household help for at least a week, and ideally, several weeks. Sometimes you just have to surrender to a messy house and let it go. And remember that your life won't always be in such wonderful chaos. My mother used to say that she would have a clean, straightened house when her babies and children were all grown up.

A flood of emotions spiral through you in the first few days of motherbaby moon time. Don't be surprised if you plunge into every emotion imaginable to the very depths of your being. What is most amazing is the overwhelming love felt for your baby. However, having just said that, also don't be surprised if you feel angry at a fussy baby who just won't stop crying. It can be extremely frustrating to care for a baby when you don't know what your baby is asking for! The passion of every cell in your body is to love and protect this tiny infant whose life is so deeply entwined with you.

Don't be surprised if fear washes over you from time to time at the very responsibility of caring for this vulnerable baby. You may feel anxiety and a loss of control. This is a time when it is important to have another person with you who can help ground you. Deep breathing and positive words can be just the recipe for helping you to calm down. If you feel as if you are spiraling into a panic, call your midwife for support. Perhaps she can talk you through your feelings.

Many women are sad at no longer being pregnant. They miss the baby's movements, or may feel that it was safer for the baby to be inside instead of outside in the outer world. If your birth didn't go as planned, emotional healing may take days, weeks, or even years. Take as much time as you need to fully experience all of your emotions during this time.

You may find that you desire to talk about your birthing experience, especially with your midwife or those who attended you. I find it interesting that most women wish to know what their behavior during labor was like from an outside perspective. It is important to tell your story and ask questions of those who were with you.

Talking through the experience helps you to integrate the process into your rational self.

Your emotions may peak at around three days after birth. Tears may flow, as it is not uncommon for new mothers to feel emotionally and physically exhausted. Hang on through the bumpy ride, as this intensity is usually temporary. Babies often have an emotional release around the second day too. I often think that people mistake this fussiness for being hungry. Sometimes you both just end of up crying together and why not? You both have come through a tremendous journey; one of great enormous change. Of course, there is a feeling of exhilaration and curiosity, but also, understandably, a sense of loss of the closeness that once was. Once again, ask for help if you are not able to bring yourself back into equilibrium, or if your baby is unable to be consoled.

Yes, great joy, feeling proud, and love from the bottom of your heart, can be felt along with fear, sadness, panic, and anxiety. This all is normal. It is yin and yang. With great joy comes great pain. With great love comes great fear. The responsibility is tremendous.

There are so many decisions to make regarding care for your baby. Look back to the intuition chapter and be sure to focus on your deep intuitive ways of knowing. Remember to trust the process of accessing your intuition and the culmination of all of your senses.

You will need the first week or so just to balance your extreme emotions while at the same time healing physically. And all of this with undoubtedly a lack of sleep! Take your time with the process.

Ruth Anne tells us about her experience with her first baby.

What a whirlwind of a time that was. I couldn't believe how I felt like a mother lion. I felt fierce in the protection of my baby! I felt as though instinct was taking over my body. It was a little scary actually. I'm glad I had a home birth because I would have gone berserk if strangers [medical workers] were near my baby. At home I was able to be in seclusion for a few days; just my husband, baby and me. I laugh now at the intensity of emotions I felt. But it was real for me in the moment.

Of course family and friends will be excited to greet the new baby and wish you well. Having visitors can be exhausting, so be careful. I recommend that families set visiting times, say 7:00-8:00 p.m. For the first few days stay in bed in your pajamas. Visitors tend to not stay as long if you appear to be resting. Resist the urge to entertain them. Like Ruth Anne, I have known other families that go into seclusion for a few days and do not allow any visitors. Pay attention to your need for protection from illness. If there has been a flu or cold epidemic going around your area it makes perfect sense to keep others away. Be clear with respect to your expectations and people will understand.

Also, make sure whomever is taking care of you is also taking care of himself/herself. I have seen fathers and partners work themselves into oblivion the first few days. Anyone who is emotionally close to you and the baby will also need his or her own time for integrating the new family norm. Truly, a community of helpers is a gift to the new family. In many communities there are postpartum doula services or mother's helpers who can provide much needed household help if you don't have family or friends nearby to help.

In *Rediscovering Birth,* social anthropologist of birth, Sheila Kitzinger writes,

> The pattern of seclusion of mother and baby, and their nurturing by women close to them, is found all over the world. It is commonly forty days, a

period in which a woman is exempt from her usual tasks and receives nourishing food and support. Traditionally, it has been an important factor both for the survival of the newborn and for the "tuning in" and emotional bonding of mother and baby, and remains the ritual ideal in many cultures (Kitzinger, 2000, p. 226).

Along with your emotions your body will be healing physically after the birth and there are a few aspects that must be attended to. You will bleed for the first few days after the birth. At first the blood, called lochia, will be similar to a heavy period. It is best to wear overnight, long sanitary napkins at this time. I have found that if you put one up near the back of your underwear and the other up the front it really cuts down on leakage. Some mothers like to wear urinary incontinence pads, which look like disposable diapers, for the first few days. If you are opposed to disposable products use a cloth about the size of a hand-towel and later when the flow slows, use wash-clothes. Tampons are not recommended as they could irritate tender vaginal tissue.

After two days or so the bright red blood lessens and becomes mucousy. The red bloody mucous gradually changes to pink with some brown colored, or old blood, in the mucous. Sometimes blood clots will form, too. They range in size from a walnut-size to lemon-size and look like liver.

One sign that you might be doing too much is if the bright red bleeding subsides and then returns. This often will happen when a mother lifts something too heavy, walks up and down steps, or gets exhausted. This is your uterus asking you to slow down. It needs time to heal where the placenta was attached. Our uteri are rather bossy, and it is a good thing they are! They are trying to protect us from ourselves!

Your flow should smell earthy, like a typical period. Signs that there may be a problem are flow smelling like rotting flesh, extreme uterine cramping or tenderness, or a fever. These are all signs that there may be some retained placenta or a uterine infection. Call your midwife immediately if you experience any of these signs.

You may have strong menstrual-like cramps after your birth, especially if this is not your first baby. Sometimes the after-cramps feel more intense than contractions of labor! The good news is that this prevents you from bleeding more than necessary. If the sensation is too intense you might like to try the herb cramp bark,

Viburnum opulus. Make a tea with one teaspoon dried cramp bark per cup of water or take a half a teaspoon of tincture. This herb takes the edge off strong cramps. Cramps are stronger during nursing because of the release of oxytocin, which brings on milk and also contracts the uterus. Concentrate on the baby and breathe through strong cramps. They generally lessen and by a few days are completely gone. Not only are these cramps reducing bleeding they also are aiding in reducing your uterus to its prepregnant size.

Isn't it amazing that your uterus grows to the shape of a watermelon and then returns to the shape of a pear? This process, called involution, takes two to three weeks. In many cultures uterine massage is given daily for several days after birth.

In Malaysia, a specially trained masseur comes every day to knead the mother's abdomen. In Europe and North America, friction and kneading were popular until early this [20th] century. To ease aching joints, Jicarillo Indian women in Mexico have their bodies massaged with a rubbing lotion made from the leaves and seeds of boiled angelpod. After each of her twenty postnatal massages, a Mayan woman has her abdomen tied with a supportive sash, just as she did during her pregnancy (Dunham, 1991, p. 128).

The first days, and sometimes weeks, after your birth are also important for giving your bottom time to heal. Even if you did not tear, your bottom will probably be sensitive from all of the hard work it did. You might want to take a sitz bath in healing herbs. A sitz bath is a shallow bath, usually about 3-4" deep that just covers your bottom. Here is my favorite recipe for a postpartum sitz bath.

Granny Janny Motherbaby Moon Time
Sitz Bath

2 parts comfrey root

2 parts comfrey leaf

1 part plantain leaf

1 part calendula flowers

1 part sea salt

(Check the resource list for information on purchasing
Granny Janny Herbs.)

Make a strong infusion, strain, and place infusion in shallow bath water. You can also immerse sanitary napkins in the infusion and then place on your bottom. Chill the sanitary napkin first if you prefer cold on your bottom.

If you have a perineal tear make a special effort to stay in bed as much as possible for the first week. Keep your legs together, and no climbing stairs or sitting cross-legged. This will encourage your tender tissues to heal while receiving the best possible blood flow.

As you spend the first few days just sitting and holding your baby pay attention to your body, especially your neck. Many new mothers get what I call "baby neck syndrome" which is stiffness and soreness from looking down so much at the baby. Make sure that you rotate your head in circles and stretch your neck often. Stretch all of your body often and try not to stay in one position too long. Move before you hurt!

Hopefully, you know a massage therapist who will come to your house to give you and your baby a massage. For you, a massage can help melt away the achiness you most likely will feel after you have given birth. Babies also benefit from a gentle massage. How wonderful it is for a baby to begin life on earth knowing the healing power of touch!

If your baby's skin gets dry and starts to peel you can massage oil into the skin, or you can use the same above mentioned herbs in the Motherbaby Moon Time Sitz bath for a healing baby bath. Calendula flower oil is also nice for baby's tender skin. Your baby may get pimply looking spots on her/his cheeks. Just leave them alone and they will go away in a few days. This is called milia and is caused by sebaceous glands opening and producing oil.

Pay attention to whether or not your baby urinates in the first day or so. Before the milk comes in the baby urinates a small amount so it can be difficult to tell, especially if you are using disposable diapers. You can put a piece of toilet paper on the diaper in order to make sure there is wetness. After your milk comes in your baby should saturate at least six to eight cloth diapers per 24-hour period. You can tell that your baby is getting enough fluids when the urine is rather clear or slightly straw colored. If the urine is concentrated, dark yellow in color and smells strongly, be sure to nurse more often. Also, make sure that you yourself are drinking enough fluids!

For the first day your baby isn't able to regulate her temperature. Be sure to dress her/him a layer warmer than what you are wearing. After the first day dress the baby similar to how you are dressed. Some families like to keep the baby's head covered at all times for several weeks. My Chinese friend says that babies' ears need to be covered so that wind won't get into the head. If it does, she warns, the wind can't get out of the head and can cause headaches and earaches.

With delayed cord cutting, jaundice is hardly ever an issue. If your baby were to be jaundiced in the first 24 hours you would need to contact your health care provider immediately. This would be a sign of blood incompatibility, which requires medical attention. If your baby becomes jaundiced after the first 24 hours the yellowing will peak at 3-5 days and then gradually subside. Most often this after-twenty-four-hours type of jaundice will resolve with extra nursing and a bit of exposure to the sun if available. Be sure to nurse often as the bilirubin, (the yellowness under the skin) is excreted by attaching to protein.

Other signs that would need immediate medical attention are inconsolable high-pitched screaming or crying, lethargy and weakness, high temperature, elevated respiration rates, jitteriness, or blueness. These are uncommon, but just be aware that they are a possibility.

Minor problems that may arise are diaper rash, heat rash, thrush, colic, and cradle cap. Diaper rashes are an annoyance and painful for baby. By changing the diaper often these rashes can often be avoided. Wash your baby's bottom at each change and use gentle soaps.

Carefully clean all of the folds and creases and let the bottom air dry whenever possible. (Watch out for little boys urinating like a water fountain!) Calendula salves are effective for coating the bottom and healing any irritations. Granny Janny Green Goop salve is also healing for sore bottoms. Check the remedies chapters for how to make these salves.

Heat rashes are caused by over heating and look like tiny raised red spots. Cool off the baby and the living space if possible. However, don't blow a fan directly on a baby. Loosely dress the baby in soft cotton or simply let the baby go naked for a while. If the baby is moist and sticky pat the skin dry with a soft cloth. Be sure to dry off the creases around the baby's pudgy neck, arms, and legs.

Thrush happens when a baby has an overgrowth of yeast. You will notice white patches on the tongue or a flat red rash on the bottom. Get some acidophilus from the pharmacy and make a paste and paint it on the entire mouth. Acidophilus is a friendly bacterium that halts the overgrowth of yeast. Yeast can't grow in the cold so you could also apply ice to the rash. Yeast overgrows on sugar so check your diet and eliminate, or greatly reduce, sugars in your diet. If thrush is bothering your baby you may want to visit your health care provider for further advice.

Breastfeeding

How amazing is it that your breasts will provide sole physical, emotional, and spiritual nourishment for your baby for several months after birth? I love the wisewoman words of Elizabeth Davis in her book *Heart and Hands: A Midwife's Guide to Pregnancy and Birth*,

It is nature's design that by giving birth, a woman learns to release her inhibitions and trust her body. This is key to a successful breastfeeding experience. Disapproving relatives or unsolicited advice may, however, interfere with maternal instincts. Breastfeeding is an intimate act between mother and baby, and so requires privacy, especially in the beginning... Orgasmic breastfeeding is more than just an intriguing concept; it's a reality for many women. The term 'orgasmic' connotes the ability to engage oneself fully in an endeavor, to respond and let go completely. Thus it is in nursing and caring for a baby (Davis, 1997, p.180).

Yes, breastfeeding is a sensual experience. Oxytocin, the "love hormone" is once again released during breastfeeding just as it is during labor and sexual intercourse. Oxytocin is all about relationships and keeping a close personal connection with the ones we love. That's why breastmilk is not just about food nourishment. It comforts and calms, too. Oxytocin stimulates the let-down of milk, and the hormone prolactin stimulates the breasts to make milk. Together the two hormones, along with frequent nursing, make for ample amounts of creamy mother's milk.

Science can not duplicate human breast milk. Strawberry flavored synthetic vitamins are to a fresh strawberry as baby formula is to breastmilk. There is no comparison. As Janet Tamaro writes in her book, *So That's What They Are For: Breastfeeding Basics,*

> Breastmilk isn't just food. It's actually closer to unstructured, living tissue (like blood) than it is to food. Because breastmilk is full of white blood cells, antibodies, vitamins, water, protein, hormones, growth factors, and even ingredients that kill bacteria and viruses, breastmilk is capable of doing for babies on the outside what nutrients fed through the placenta do on the inside. It offers the perfect balance of everything a baby needs to develop physically and neurologically (Tamaro, 1996, p 27).

Continue to eat a rainbow of highly nutritious foods everyday. It takes quite a bit of energy to make breastmilk, so be sure you are eating high quality food. Avoid foods that have been sprayed with pesticides, herbicides, and other chemicals as much as possible. Gina Soloman, M.D., M.P.H., a senior scientist at the Natural Resources Defense Council (NRDC) and an expert on pollution in mother's milk, advises women to drink lots of water, eat organic food, avoid fish high in mercury such as swordfish, shark, and tuna steaks. If you eat locally grown fish she says to be sure there are no advisories against it (Solomon, 2001, p.2).

"For the first few days your breasts will give colostrum which is thick, and is low in fat and carbohydrates, and high in proteins. Colostrum is also high in antibodies and protects your baby from many outside microbes. These immunities protect your baby from illnesses that you are immune to" (La Leche League, 1996, p. 350). The baby only receives a few drops of colostrum at each feeding. Gradually your breasts switch from colostrum to thinner breastmilk. While waiting for your milk to come in your baby gets her/his energy by metabolizing a special fat, called brown fat, that is stored in the baby's body during the last few weeks of pregnancy. This is nature's design to provide for her/him while giving the body a chance to gradually learn the work of digesting vast amounts of milk.

As your colostrum switches to milk you may notice that you feel a little feverish and that your breasts are engorged. This is normal and will gradually subside. Engorgement does not mean that your breasts are filled with that much milk. Actually, vessels swelling as they prepare for the process of making milk cause the engorgement. Sometimes mothers are concerned when the engorgement lessens. They feel that they are not making enough milk. This couldn't be further from the truth. You will make plenty of milk no matter what your breast size.

When your baby begins to nurse you may notice a strong tingly, prickly sensation. This is called the let-down reflex and happens when the 15-20 milk ducts that you have in each breast relax and release milk. You may or may not leak between feedings.

If your nipples are intensely painful when your baby begins to nurse, or if they are cracking, try changing the baby's mouth position a bit or move the baby's body into a slightly different angle. Many mothers have found that if they keep the baby's belly touching their belly the pain subsides or greatly lessens. In other words, keep the baby's belly completely parallel with your body. If you still have trouble call your local La Leche League group. Use a comfrey salve on your nipples, or let your nipples be open to the fresh air. Don't give up! Find the positive support from others. Breathe through the pain and know it will subside.

How often should you nurse your baby? Breastmilk digests quicker than formula or cow's milk so you will need to nurse often, sometimes every hour or so. Formula fed babies are fed every 3-4 hours. Times between breastfeeding will often stretch from 1 1/2 to 2 hours. There is no need to be aware of clock time. Rather, pay attention to your baby's cues. Some signs that your baby wishes to nurse are sucking on her/his hand, rooting (moving the head towards anything that the cheek touches), fussiness, or other ways unique to your baby.

Try out other nursing positions besides sitting and cradling the baby. You could try lying on your side with your baby facing you. A comfy rocking chair is also wonderful while nursing. Before you begin nursing make sure that you have a glass of water with you, and that you are very comfortable before the baby latches on. This is important since you may be sitting in one position for quite a while.

Be sure that you nurse on both sides for a few minutes. Some mothers consciously start with one breast at one feeding and the other breast at the next feeding. Most often the baby will linger on the second breast. Altering the breast your baby lingers on will even out the amount of stimulation to each breast and keep your supply equal. With time you will find the rhythm and patterns that work for both of you.

One of the joys of breastfeeding is that the baby's bowel movements don't smell offensive at all. Usually they are rather sweet smelling. The first bowel movement is called meconium. It is thick and looks like tar. Watch out because if it dries on the baby's bottom it is hard to get off. If this happens put some oil on the bottom and let it soak in before trying to wash it off. Meconium gradually transitions into a green color, which in turn leads to a mustard yellow color. White curds may also be found in the runny mustard colored bowel movements. The mustard yellow color stays until your baby eats solid food.

If the bowel movement is green it may be a sign that you have too much sugar in your diet or that the baby is not feeling well. You may want to contact your health care provider if this happens. Some babies have a bowel movement every time they feed, some once a day, and others every few days. In general your baby will follow his/her own pattern.

Breastfeeding is convenient. Breastmilk is always warm, always right with you, and there is no clean up. Breastmilk keeps the baby's skin and hair smelling sweet. But for many women, the best part of breastfeeding is the closeness of motherbaby; the utter bliss and interconnectedness felt by both. The chemistry of breastfeeding alters the physiology of both mother and baby to bring on a deep sense of relaxation and calmness. Breastfeeding without a doubt brings a mother to the dream world and helps her to relate to the essence of her newborn.

Language of Babies

The natural mothering path invites you to slow down to the baby's pace and helps you to pay attention to your baby in a deep way. In the wonderful booklet, *Being With Babies—What Babies are Teaching Us*, author Wendy Anne McCarty, Ph.D., tells us, "Babies are exquisitely sensitive to and impacted by our shifts in our attention. Babies are so fluid and merge with us so readily, that they are deeply affected by the changes in our focus, as well as changes in our emotions" (McCarty, 2000, p.18).

Babies have a purity of expression. Emotions are expressed through facial expressions, crying, pretending to be asleep, a speeding of heart or respiration rates, or other individual ways. In general, babies are easily overwhelmed, startled, or scared. Especially during motherbaby moon time protect yourselves from too much activity and outside influences. Take time to get to know one another!

Scientists, who research the brains of infants find that the delta and theta EEG ranges are predominant. This means that babies are in a kind of deep thought and dream world. These states are associated with restorative and regenerative processes, deep creativity, active learning and acute observations.

Attachment Parenting

Observe your baby's cues carefully and soon you will be fluent in the motherbaby language without words. To stay in touch and aware with the language of their babies many mothers practice what is now called attachment parenting. The guiding principle of attachment parenting is being responsive to your baby's language. To accomplish this a mother needs to be close to her baby at all times. Thus she carries the baby throughout the day in a sling or baby carrier. The baby moves with the rhythm of life much as she/he did in utero. The baby's senses are alive with the love of her/his mother. The baby listens to the mother's heart, smells her sweet milk and flows with the pace of the day.

In general, attachment parenting includes:

♥ Babywearing—(This phrase was coined by John and Martha Sears who are authors and proponents of attachment parenting.) Babywearing means that a baby is carried for several weeks after birth either in a sling, front pack or back pack. "The physical connection with the mother is considered so essential that in some African cultures the cloth that attaches the baby to its mother's back is called the 'placenta' (Kitzinger, 2000, p.230).

♥ No separation of Motherbaby—Mother and baby are considered as one person for several weeks after birth. This is the fourth season of pregnancy. The constant closeness of the baby to mother creates security for both. Hence, the phrase motherbaby. Both of you really are dependent upon one another. This means staying close both night and day.

♥ Co-sleeping—The baby sleeps next to the mother either in the same bed or in a bed extender. Oftentimes both mother and baby sleep more soundly when sleeping together. When they are together they are motherbaby. When apart they become mother and baby; if they are too far apart their senses go looking for one another.

♥ Intuitive knowledge—Most importantly, attachment parenting means being aware of your intuitive messages. Your intuition will guide you as you listen to your baby's cues.

♥ Demand breastfeeding—No need to pay attention to the clock. Simply breastfeed whenever the baby wants or needs to. As mentioned earlier, breast milk digests quickly. Pay attention to baby cues and you will understand when your baby needs to nurse.

♥ Respond without delay to baby's cues—By spending lots of time with your baby you will soon learn to understand your baby's different cries, facial expressions, and energy levels. These are the languages of your baby. When you respond immediately to your baby you are encouraging trust and your baby will feel secure. Imagine how you would feel if your husband or partner ignored you every time you spoke. You would not be very happy and would probably feel unloved and not respected. Why should your baby feel any different?

There are many books published now that are entirely devoted to the concepts of attachment parenting, and natural mothering (The two terms are often thought of as one and the same). I have included many of them in the reference list at the end of this book. You might want to read them or share them with family members and friends who may be concerned about your mothering style.

Circumcision

If your baby is a boy the question of whether or not to circumcise will come up. Circumcision is a surgical procedure that removes some of the foreskin from the penis. The foreskin is skin that extends from the shaft of the penis, covers the end of the penis, and folds in on itself to come to a small opening in the end. After a few years, often around age three, the intact foreskin retracts back to expose the end of the penis.

The American Academy of Pediatrics has stated that there are no proven medical reasons for circumcision and they discourage it. Nonetheless, in 1994, 64 percent of baby boys were still circumcised in the United States (Ray, 1997, p.2). In many other countries circumcision is unheard of and not practiced even when requested unless for medical reasons.

So why perform a routine surgery when it is unnecessary? Rituals are hard to change; especially ones that are emotionally charged. Let's look at some reasons parents have decided to circumcise their baby boy.

- ♥ We want our son to look like his dad.
- ♥ An uncircumcised penis looks gross.
- ♥ It is the will of God.
- ♥ Uncircumcised penises are not clean.
- ♥ It is just what people do.

Here is a list of reasons parents have decided not to circumcise.

- ♥ Nature intended the foreskin to be there for protection. It has a purpose.
- ♥ I could not torture my baby boy like that.
- ♥ We are Jewish. We had a symbolic circumcision as I could not put my baby through that pain.
- ♥ Circumcision goes against my mothering instincts to protect my baby.

- ♥ Circumcising for cleanliness reasons is like removing the tonsils of a newborn because he might get a sore throat later in life.

- ♥ My son can make that decision for himself later on if he wants to.

- ♥ I have heard that a man has a more satisfying sex life if he is not circumcised.

- ♥ Gosh, I wouldn't dream of circumcising my baby girl, so why should it be different for a boy?

I talked with five boys, ages ten through twenty-one, who are not circumcised. They unanimously were grateful to their parents that the surgery was not done to them. (I noticed that many of them were rocking, or had their hands near their groin when talking about it.) None of them had ever had any medical problems related to being intact. They also mentioned other boys, who were circumcised, had never teased them. In fact, one of the boys had mentioned that a circumcised friend of his was angry when he discovered that he had been circumcised and was never told.

Linda, a mother of seven says,

We don't circumcise. We don't feel like it is natural. It is painful for the child. It is totally pointless. I think one of the arguments for it was to prevent infections. If you leave the foreskin alone you shouldn't have any problems. My boys have never had any problems. My son has mentioned that he is grateful he is not circumcised. He doesn't try to hide the fact that he is not circumcised. He has made comments before, wondering why any body would do that.

Lorene tells us her story of circumcising her first baby boy and not the others.

The next day after he was born they wake me up at 6:00 am and say it is time to do the circumcision. My husband and his brother are circumcised so I thought, well, ok, that is just what you do. I had never heard of anyone not circumcising. So they took him away. He came back and he was in a deep sleep and shock for a long time. I can't tell you how badly I feel about that. Now that I have other boys who are not circumcised you can see why the foreskin is there. Circumcision is male genital mutilation. Well, I am here to tell you I have seen both [circumcised penis and intact penises] and circumcision is cruel. There is no reason for this. People need to be educated about this. I was so mad when my second son was born and the pediatrician asked me three times if I was sure I didn't want to circumcise him. I was so mad I wrote a letter to his boss. I wanted them to know what he was doing to me and to other people. He badgered me about it. But he didn't give any information on why it should have been done.

Vaccinations

You will undoubtedly need to do a lot of homework before making a decision on whether or not to vaccinate. This decision can really be made easier if you already have a strong natural health care philosophy. As usual, when making decisions, you will need to look at your individual baby, family lifestyle, and general health. Gather as much information as possible from both sides of the issue, and make your decision based on knowledge and your intuition. You may feel as if you are being coerced or bullied into vaccinating your baby by medical providers, family, friends, and schools. Stand strong within yourself. Remember that you are responsible for the care your baby. If you decide not to vaccinate your baby it may help to know that many parents following the natural path are not vaccinating.

Pros and Cons of Vaccinating

Just what are vaccinations and how do they work? In an online letter, Philip Incao, M.D. writes, "Until recently, the 'mechanism of actions' of vaccinations was always understood to be simply that they cause an increase in antibody levels (titers) against a specific disease antigen (bacterium or virus), thus preventing 'infection' with that bacterial or viral antigen" (Incao, 1999, p.1).

Recently science has increased its knowledge of the immune system to understand that there is much more to the immune process than was earlier thought. The immune system is actually composed of two functional branches or compartments, which may work together in a mutually cooperative way *or* a mutually antagonistic way. Which way it works depends on the individual person and her/his general health.

One part of the immune system is called the humoral immune system that produces antibodies in the blood circulation. The humoral immune system recognizes antigens or foreign bodies such as viruses and bacteria, creates antibodies, and sends out a message to the other part of the immune system called the cellular or cell-mediated immune system. The humoral part of the immune system is what is activated after a vaccination. In theory, everyone who is vaccinated should aquire antibodies against the disease. There are problems with accepting this theory of immunization after vaccination, some of which are:

♥ There is no guarantee that everyone vaccinated will be immune to the disease; For example, "the New England Journal of Medicine published a study revealing that the pertussis vaccine 'failed to give...protection against the disease.' In fact, more than 80 percent of cases in a recent epidemic occurred in children who had received regular doses of the shot" (Global Vaccine Institute, 2004, p.1).

♥ We have always been told that breastfeeding gives a baby immunity from diseases that the mother has had. If this is true why are breastfed infants encouraged to get their vaccinations on the same schedule as those who are not?

♥ Vaccination gives a false sense of security. For example, The International Medical Observer states that " a new strain of measles resistant to vaccine has been discovered" (Global Vaccine Institute, 2004, p.4).

Of major concern are the effects of vaccination on the cell-mediated part of the immune system that eliminates the antigens or foreign bodies. White blood cells that are found in the thymus, tonsils, adenoids, spleen, lymph nodes, and lymph system, go out and find the antigens and destroy them by digesting them or ending the antigen's life by chemical processes. This process is known as "the acute inflammatory response." During this response the individual will feel one or more of these signs of inflammation: fever, rash, increased mucous, achiness in joints and muscles, headaches, redness and swelling in infected area, irritability or lethargy.

Looking at the immune system from a holistic perspective one can understand how difficult it could be for the entire system after a vaccination. Theoretically it is possible that the cell-mediated response might become confused and over stimulated because of a vaccine. Research has shown that concurrent with our mass immunization program we have seen a rise of allergies, attention deficit disorder, autism, asthma, and other neuroimmune dysfunction (Reagan, 2001, p.3).

Side effects of vaccinations are usually allergic, or auto-immune inflammatory reactions, caused by the shift of the immune system's reactivity from the cell-mediated response to the humoral response. Modern medicine is just beginning to recognize this.

Ideally, a vaccination includes just enough of the disease antigen to stimulate the humoral immune system but not enough to cause the disease. In other words, the humoral part of the immune system makes antibodies without stimulating the cell-mediated part of the immune system. Herein lies the enormous unanswered question with mass vaccinations. Lisa Reagan writes in her *Mothering Magazine* article, Show Us the Science: An exclusive Mothering Report on the Second International Public Conference of the National Vaccine Information Center,

> Public health, like individual health, is not measured solely by an absence of infectious disease. And so one of the great unanswered questions in medicine today is: has the mass use of multiple vaccines in early childhood, when the brain and immune systems are developing at their most rapid rate, been a major co-factor in the broad-based brain and immune dysfunctions seen in so many young children and young adults today (Reagan, 2001, p.3)?

Here are the words of Ruth Anne, a natural mother who speaks of why she chose not to vaccinate her four children,

> *I choose not to vaccinate for several reasons. First and foremost, I believe that there is a lot of false security with vaccinations. I mean, how would I know that they were immune? I was always bothered by the strong reactions that I saw some of my friend's babies go through. Some of them didn't seem healthy again for a long time afterward: just in time for them to get their next vaccination. My intuition told me that vaccines actually weaken the body.*

Ruth Anne continues,

> *My health care belief system is first and foremost to stay as healthy as possible. We always try to live a healthy lifestyle by eating organic whole foods, drinking a lot of water, sleeping as much as needed, getting fresh air and exercise and staying happy and stress free. I know the illnesses are horrible that vaccines were made to prevent. I wouldn't want anyone's child to go through those illnesses. But it is not as easy as they make it sound. I know a person who acquired polio from*

having a vaccine. This is a hard choice, but I would rather strive for keeping my family healthy and not vaccinate, instead of vaccinating and take the chance they would have a strong reaction to the vaccine. There is no long-term research on the safety of vaccines and the side affects can be horrendous.

And finally, studies have shown that as families improve their living conditions through increased hygiene, better nutrition, clean water, fresh air, feeling connected and loved within a family and community that the rate of life threatening diseases go down.

~Six~

Where Will Your Birthing Nest Be?

As always, use all of your senses when deciding where you plan to give birth. The bottom line is that you need to give birth wherever you feel the safest and most supported. When your birthing environment is just right your inhibitions will go out the door and will allow you to be your authentic self in labor. Contractions will flow freely when a laboring woman is comfy in her birthing nest. Where will your nest be?

Thoughts you may want to consider when deciding where you will labor and birth are:

- ♥ Where will I feel the safest when I give birth?
- ♥ What environment do I wish to be in when in labor and giving birth?
- ♥ Do I believe I have the power and wisdom to give birth on my own?
- ♥ Will I feel safer with technology around me?
- ♥ Am I deeply afraid to go through the process?
- ♥ Do I feel that laboring and birthing naturally are important for my baby?

- ❤ Do I feel that laboring and birthing naturally are important for myself?

- ❤ Is labor and birth a medical event?

- ❤ Is the process of labor and delivery a natural life experience?

- ❤ Is labor and birth a sensual, sexual experience?

- ❤ Am I afraid of death?

- ❤ Am I afraid of hard work?

- ❤ Do I truly feel that my baby and myself would be safer in the hospital or birth center?

- ❤ Am I attracted to a water birth? (Many hospitals will not allow delivery in the water.)

- ❤ Am I willing to pay a midwife out of pocket for a home birth?

Sara Wickham, midwife, researcher and midwifery lecturer writes in her booklet, *What's right for me: Making decisions in pregnancy and birth,*

> Choosing the place where you will give birth is one of the most important decisions you will make. The environment you are in while you labor and give birth can have a profound effect on you. This effect can be positive or negative and it can influence your and your baby's entire experience. The most important issue is that you are totally

comfortable with the place in which you will give birth. More and more women today are choosing to give birth in their own homes. Part of the reason for this is the discovery that, even when women's "rational" brains think they are safer in the hospital, the more instinctive parts of their brain perceive it [the hospital] as an unsafe and threatening environment. Experiencing this situation—which also occurs with birthing animals that stop their labor and move on with the rest of their herd when they smell danger—can cause women's bodies to go "out of labor." This may then lead to potentially unnecessary interventions in the birth process (Wickham, 2002, p.28-29).

When choosing where your birthing nest will be it is also extremely important to carefully choose a birth attendant whose philosophies about birth, and health care in general, are similar to yours. The following paradigms, written by Robbie Davis-Floyd, a medical/cultural anthropologist, are central to the care a birth attendant gives. These paradigms are an adaptation from the Robbie's book, *Birth as a American Rite of Passage*, and are found in Anne Frye's book, *Holistic Midwifery: Volume I—Care During Pregnancy.*

Characteristics of the Technocratic Model of Care

Basic Principle = Separation

1. Mechanization of the body
2. Isolation and objectification of the patient
3. A focus on curing disease, repairing, dysfunction
4. Aggressive, interventionist approach to diagnosis and treatment
5. Alienation of practitioner from patient
6. Supervaluation of technology
7. Hierarchical organization of the patient as subordinate to practitioner and institution
8. Authority and responsibility inherent in the practitioner

Characteristics of the Holistic Model of Care

Basic Principle = Connection

1. Views the body as an energy system interlinked with other energy systems
2. Insistence that total healing requires attention to the body-mind-spirit-emotions-family-community-environment
3. A focus on creating and maintaining health and well-being

4. Nurturing, relational approach to diagnosis and treatment

5. Essential unity of practitioner and client

6. Respect for the value of inner knowing

7. Technology at the service of the individual

8. Later, webbed organization-networking

9. Authority and responsibility inherent in the individual (Frye, 1995, p.2-3).

In general, those working in the hospital setting follow the technocratic model, and midwives attending home birth follow the holistic model. This, of course, is a generalization. Sometimes midwives attending home births can work well within the technocratic model and nurse-midwives and doctors can work within the holistic framework while in a hospital setting. Ask many questions when interviewing birth attendants and find a care provider who has beliefs and philosophies that align with yours. Share with possible birth attendants that you will be following a natural mothering path. Choose your attendant carefully.

Giving birth in the comfort of one's own home is a viable option that many natural mothers choose. After all, babies have been born at home from the beginning of human time and the world is plenty populated!

Jill Cohen, midwife and associate editor of *Midwifery Today* magazine writes,

> It has only been in the last century that out-of-home birthing became the norm, a change engineered by ambitious men during a time when it was believed best to bring the natural world under control. What resulted in the birthing world was a surge into the hospital. It started with a fad, developed into a sign of prestige, then became pervasive when fear took over. With it came the inevitable spiral of cause and effect; the more intervention was introduced, the more it was needed, until birth was no longer recognizable as a natural process in human experience. Instead, it had been orchestrated into an assembly line procedure complete with time constraints, quotas, indifferent workers, procedures manuals, and loss of individual rights and autonomy (Cohen, 1999, p.1).

Since the 1920s we have been hoodwinked into believing that the hospital is the safest place to birth. The transition from home to hospital births happened when there was an insurgence of technological gadgets and with them, a displaced sense of trust on outward mechanisms instead of internal knowing. Because of technology, we have been so removed from nature, natural process, and hard work that we now believe we need to be rescued from the simple, but intense, experience of giving birth. Our culture, in general, also believes that technology has rescued us from the hard physical work of everyday living.

Other issues that surface are not wanting to take responsibility for health care, and fear. Considering labor and birth, women can be saturated with fear of the unknown, and the intensity of labor. If you avoid intense life experiences before being pregnant it certainly can make the idea of giving birth daunting. As a whole these are cultural issues that need to be considered.

I remember my Grandma telling me stories about how proud women were when they first got electricity. Along with that came washers and dryers, stoves, irons, etc. They believed these appliances would make their lives easier. They also believed that going to the hospital to birth would make their lives easier and their births safer.

When I was growing up I remember when many of the farmwomen in our community cooked on wood stoves. It was too hot in the summer for everyone to cook over a fire so they took turns cooking and shared foods with other families in the neighborhood. When they washed clothes by hand they did it as a community project. They gathered herbs and made their own medicines for the wintertime. These women worked together in all aspects of their lives. But when the women started getting their appliances, working together as a community stopped. That's how it was with birthing too. My Grandma said, "In one generation women forgot how to have their babies." She always believed it was a great loss for women when they gave up birthing their babies in their own beds, began washing their clothes in a machine, and started depending on a doctor for their medicine. I believe it too. Technology has not freed people from hard work and the chores of living. In fact there is no freedom from the chores of living. You just have to do it. And that includes birthing your babies, too.

Make no doubt about it; birthing your baby is hard work. No one can do it for you, or rescue you from labor. Even women who have planned cesareans have to recover from major abdominal surgery. There is no way out without some work on your part. The final destination has deeper meaning when you have to work hard to get there. So, strongly consider whether or not you are willing to go to the depth of your being to birth your baby. At a home birth there is no way out; you have to do the work yourself. While in a hospital setting there are interventions to "rescue" you from the process, but there are consequences nonetheless.

Lorene tells the story of her hospital birth and the confusion it caused her by being in an environment that was less than optimal for her.

*It was a typical hospital delivery. When I arrived at the hospital they put me in a wheel chair and wheeled me up to the room and made me stay in the bed. Then they put the (baby) monitor around me. I didn't know that I didn't have to do those things at that time. I just went with it. I told them that I wanted a natural birth because my mother had had a natural birth with my brother. I wanted to have a natural delivery but, my gosh, when you are strapped into a bed you beg for it. "Please give me drugs. Please give me drugs!" It hurts so much more when you can't move and you can't do what your body tells you to do. With my other births, in a birth center and at home, I birthed so easy. I am made to birth. **I am made to birth**. That is what makes me so mad about the whole thing.*

Someone like me births so easily, and if they do all of that to me, that is why it happens to everybody else. There is no reason for all of this stuff they do to you in the hospital.

So I get in there...I have never seen the facilities. I was with a nurse I had never seen before. I was not comfortable with the situation. All of the pretty birthing rooms were busy, so I was shoved into a delivery room. The anesthesiologist said it was too late for an epidural so they gave me Demoral [meperidine] instead. My son was born soon afterwards. The second after he was born I just had weird distorted thoughts. I just thought I should keep looking at him because if he dies, and I don't remember what he looks like, I will feel really bad. The second he came out of me they took him away from me and put him on a little platform. My baby was screaming at the top of his lungs. They were paying attention to me and I couldn't go over there because I was still feeling the effects of the Demerol. He kept screaming, and I felt so messed up. Every instinct that I had was messed up. So my mother went over to the baby. They [the nurses] weren't trying to make him feel comfortable. It wasn't a good situation for my baby or me. My instincts became so screwed up I couldn't figure out how to do anything. I couldn't take care of him. Once I brought him home, though, I remembered everything. I knew what to do.

Now compare Lorene's second birth story to her first. Both babies were born in the hospital, but the second time a nurse-midwife and doctor, who both believe in the holistic model of care, attended her.

When I was pregnant with my second baby I was really scared. I didn't want to have such a hard time in my life again. With my second baby I went to a midwife/doctor team that I really liked. The midwife practiced parenting like I did. She had a home birth, she didn't circumcise her son, she home-schooled her children, and was a vegetarian. She understood my parenting style; which made me feel secure with her. What she would do for herself she would do for me. The doctor was a down home kind of doctor. My second birth was totally different. I was able to follow my own instincts. I labored in public. During labor I went out with my mother to garage sales, to a restaurant, and to the post office. When I was at the post office I knew I better get to the hospital soon. So I drove to the hospital, parked my car and walked up to the second floor. When I got into my room I went to the bathroom and they were barely able to get me out of the bathroom before the baby was born. It was a vertical delivery. My husband never even made it there on time; he missed the birth. It was fantastic!

While pushing, the doctor held me up in a hanging squat. I just felt so empty; like I needed support. The midwife caught him, literally. The second he was out he went into my arms and started nursing; before the placenta was even out! He breastfed for two-hours straight. I wouldn't let any one take him away. He was born at 2:00 in the afternoon and it was 11:00 p.m. before they even took him out of my arms. They didn't even wash him. I just loved the smell of him. I didn't get to smell my first baby. That smell is just like God coming out of you. It is the ultimate; it is creation. It is so incredibly powerful.

When I was pregnant with my third baby I started learning about water births. I wanted a water birth. The hospitals would not allow anyone to birth in water in this area. So I had to go to a town that was about 40 minutes away to get the birth that I wanted. My third baby was born at a free-standing birthing center. One of the midwives put essential oils in the water and then gave me a little bottle of the oils she had used. Sometimes I get the oils out and just sniff them just to make me feel like I am there again. Again, I just made it there [to the birth center]. When my third was born I wanted to have the other kids attend the birth. I think it is important for the other kids to see their siblings being born. I prepared them by watching birth videos with them, and acting out the birth.

I really wanted a water birth. I exercise in the water and I can barely feel the effects of exercise. I feel more like a kid playing. So...my baby was born within a half-hour of getting to the birth center. It was fantastic. My mom and my dad were there watching the other children. That birth was a joyous family event.

When Loreli was asked how she came to the decision to birth her babies at home she said,

I just didn't think there was any other choice for me. I always knew that when I had children I would birth them at home and not go where people go when they are ill. It seems to me that the way babies come into the world is important. A birth at home has a different vibration than in the hospital. It was just so natural for me to have a home birth. I couldn't imagine strangers poking and prodding at me. I wanted just women around me. I thought I would want water births, but I didn't. I needed to be grounded because I am already watery and airy. I needed to feel the earth. I needed my feet on the ground. I wanted to squat. I knew I wouldn't have all of the freedom in the hospital to labor the way I needed to. I needed lots of space. People would ask me, "Aren't you afraid to birth at home?" My response was that I was afraid to birth in the hospital!

My decision to birth at home was really based on intuition. In my experience when I am in touch with my intuition I am confident. When I am confident then I can make choices that are right for me. My confidence in intuition would help me decide whether I should have tests that are often given to pregnant women. I would check in with my intuitive ways of knowing in deciding if the test was necessary. I also asked my deep self, "What do I want for my birth? What is important?" When I am listening within, the answers come to me and I can make choices without too much trouble. It becomes natural.

Linda, who birthed six of her seven children at home says,

I think that the neatest thing about home birth is that your whole family can be there when you want them there. Nobody has to go away and no one has to be subjected to strangers and the hospital's rules and regulations. You are just home. You can be exactly who you are with your baby. Home birth is a continuation of everyday life. With one of my births I remember looking out the window and focusing on the trees. It was in the fall. My midwives were such a calming presence. I felt so close to my husband. It was perfect. I couldn't think of giving birth any other way after that.

A baby that is conceived from a loving relationship is the culmination and physical manifestation of that love. That child unifies the sexual energy of the couple. I love what Naoli Vinaver, a mother and midwife from Mexico, says about her contractions in the video *Birth Day*: " I realized when I was walking towards my husband that the sensation in my womb was as if the sun wanted to burst out of my belly. If I looked at him it became very clear it was our love that was swollen inside my belly. When I looked away from him it kind of felt like pain"(Paul-Bort, 1999, video). To deepen their bond, partners need space during labor to delve into the experience without feeling inhibited.

Birth environment is so very important when one considers labor and birth as extensions of our sensual and sexual selves. *"For me giving birth is like having intercourse,"* says Ruth Anne. *"The environment is very similar. I need dim lights, warmth, and privacy to have a wonderful sexual experience. That is the same environment that I need for labor too. I knew that I couldn't make love in a hospital room with bright lights and strangers around, so why should I think I could birth my baby there?"*

Creating and guarding the birthing mother and her nest are the roles of supportive women, friends, family, doulas, and midwives. Supportive women attending you are especially important if you choose to birth in a hospital. These women surround the laboring woman with the kind of love that defines sisterhood and divine feminine energy. I once saw a video of Middle Eastern women circling around a laboring woman while they were all belly dancing. The deep connection of the divine feminine is apparent when women share their birthings and care for one another.

Ancient voices, eternal mothers, will also shine their light down upon you. This sacred, divine light can be hard to sense when florescent lights and beeping machines are all around you. Dear women, protect your birthing environment passionately. It does matter.

First impressions for a baby are important. Think carefully about what your baby's first impressions will be. Do you want your baby's first impressions to be of the warmth and love of you or beeping machines and bright lights? The environment we are born into does create the framework for our perceptions of life on earth. How do we know that this short period of time in a person's life really matters? Consider that there are many ways of knowing what is best for us. These ways of knowing can be shown to us through many different mediums: body wisdom, intuition, the wisdom of our elders, cellular memories from how our ancestors lived, and dreams.

One way that I came to understand just how important a gentle birth is was through a dream of my own birth. One night, while attending a birth, I slept while my midwifery partner sat with the laboring mother. While I slept, I dreamt of my own birth. As the dream began my mother was pushing me out. I remember the rhythmic contractions. During contractions my head felt as though I was receiving a wonderful head massage. As my head was crowning the coolness of the room left me with a curious feeling. When my head was born and my shoulders rotated I opened up an eye to see the nurse looking down towards me. I remember how she looked. This is how my Mother verified that the dream was reality. The nurse had black-horned rimmed glasses, graying hair with a bobbed haircut, a nurse's cap, and white colored clothes. There were also two other nurses who were standing back a bit, but I couldn't make out their details.

As the rest of my body was born I was shocked at how cold I felt and how quickly my body was being moved. I was upside down when I looked to see a man's face looking towards me. I was curious about his black, curly hair. That hair really stood out in my mind, and to this day I love black, curly hair. I am deeply attracted to it. While hanging upside down I remember gasping for air and feeling scared. Probably that is when the cord was cut. My guess is that it had not stopped pulsating yet. Or perhaps the ether my Mother was given inhibited my respiratory efforts. (I was born in 1959. This is a time when women were given ether just before the baby was born.) At that time the doctor turned me head up and held me in his arms. I focused on that black hair again. I wanted to let my curiosity flow but was distracted. I felt as though my chest was constricted, and I felt fear emanating in the room. I was acutely aware of emotions others in the room were feeling.

I remember how the sounds of voices were different, how there seemed to be a feeling of concern in the room. I continued to gasp for air. At the same time I was shocked to not feel my Mother's presence. I remembered the deep feelings of wanting her; I wanted the familiar. I longed for warmth, and darkness, and the sounds of her—her heartbeat and her voice. (Because of the ether my Mother was not available to me.)

Then I was placed in a warmer. I remember it felt odd to lie flat out. I didn't like the stimulation the nurses and doctor were giving me. It felt too rough. They were scared. I was scared. I didn't like any of it. My last dream memory was of an oxygen mask going on my face. The oxygen was cold too. What was up with all of this cold around me? I started to get mad. Then I took a deep gasp of air. The dream was then finished.

This dream has been a great gift to me. It reminds me that the natural path encourages no separation of motherbaby at birth. It encourages me as a midwife to remember the importance of warmth, security, and gentleness for honoring the motherbaby experience. I understand deeply that motherbaby are two people as one and that their security and safety depend upon one another. The gentle care and mindful attentiveness of the birth attendant is instrumental for the experience of motherbaby to unfold as nature intended.

Please, choose your birth attendant and place of birth carefully. Search hard for the attendant that you connect well with. You and your baby deserve to be treated with the utmost respect and dignity. There are attendants who believe in the sacredness and sanctity of birth. You may, however, need to act as a detective while finding them.

Home birth midwives, and the few doctors who attend home births, are passionate about keeping home birth a viable option. "Regardless of whatever law may be applied to the surface of women's lives, home birth is a right. In a nod to this fact, lawmakers have carefully kept their hands off this right and gone after the home birth attendant instead. Many women have had to go to great lengths to exercise their rights, however, and home birth midwives who are in the minority and sometimes practice illegally, work hard to help preserve it" (Cohen, 1999, p.1).

Given this fact you may have to search out a birth attendant who will support you and who believes in natural mothering and birthing. Good places to search are:

- ♥ La Leche League meetings
- ♥ Local food co-ops
- ♥ Birth classes (try independent classes not affiliated with hospitals)
- ♥ Yellow pages under midwives (sometimes the heading reads midwives-lay)
- ♥ Go on the internet and search for midwives (however, many midwives do not advertise on the internet so don't give up if you don't find anyone close)

While you are deciding where your birthing nest will be and who will attend you please remember this very important point. Birth almost always works and works well. For the few times it doesn't go well, we can then ask for the appropriate use of medical care. It just doesn't make sense that your body would have the wisdom to know how to grow a baby and then not be able to birth. You are about to embark on a sacred journey. Think hard about your journey and don't let fear bully you into believing that you won't be able to do it!

~Seven~

The Role of the Midwife at Labor and Birth

Midwife means "with woman." Any birth attendant who practices within the holistic model of care framework could be given the honorable name of midwife. A midwife attends to a birth with a keen eye, heart and soul. A midwife's observation skills and intuitive ways of knowing are heightened while being in the timeless space of watching and patiently waiting. A midwife is a guardian for the motherbaby and looks toward a safe passage for both of them. A midwife's role is not to control the process, but rather, to support the story of this birth, in this time and place.

In *Rediscovering Birth*, Sheila Kitzinger writes,

Midwives who attended home births always needed to adapt to the domestic environment, which they entered as guests. Family life had to go on. It was rarely just a midwife and her patient. Other children, grannies, the husband, the neighbors—all took part in the unfolding script of childbirth, and the midwife worked surrounded by a bustle of people coming and going, and sometimes the baby's father snoring on the other side of the bed (Kitzinger, 2000, p.138).

It seems as if the birth is a story waiting to be played out, and the midwife is but one character in the play. Many times the story does not make sense while in the middle of the experience, but in the end there is a greater understanding of why the process unfolded as it did. There are many lessons that we all learn from birth. Many believe, as do I, that birth is the greatest teacher. Birth is a metaphor for life and teaches us all about our deepest selves. Not only do the woman and her family learn from the experience, but the midwife learns and understands, with more depth and clarity, the mysteries of life from each birth.

Sometimes, when a birth doesn't go just as planned or hoped for, the mother may feel as if she has failed. She may feel that her body didn't/doesn't work well or that maybe she was wrong, "maybe birth shouldn't be trusted." Perhaps there are deeper life lessons for her to understand through her birthing experience. If not right now, then some time in the future, she will understand the learning that was available to her through this birthing experience. Maybe the Divine Spirit has a message for her. Given time most stories begin to make sense. The baby may also be a messenger of a deeper lesson for life. I have known babies who needed medical care and stayed in the hospital soon after birth. These babies have really brought separated extended families back together again as they rally for their new family member.

Birth is the essence of the mysterious, elemental, embodied feminine energy. This energy flows with the rhythms of life and is an inner, spiraling movement. In a natural birth, this energy can not be controlled any more than the weather. A midwife understands this and views her role as one of supporting the mother and baby while they travel together through their journey of birth. The midwife knows in her heart that authoritative behavior and interventions on her part may inhibit the true story of the birth she is attending. She stands in awe and reverence before the laboring woman and recognizes the power and beauty of the work of labor and birth.

Patience is a midwife's middle name. She knows how to wait and watch for the process to unfold. If the birthing energy becomes stagnant she can suggest ideas to encourage it to flow again. Sometimes just suggesting a change of position, a drink of juice, or for others to leave the environment is what is needed for the moment. She knows that the power of gentle touch and a gentle voice can calm frenetic energy.

The environment is very important for birthing energy to keep moving. A midwife's role is to protect this environment. "The midwife works at the intersection of time, as generation gives way to generation. In helping to make the birth space, she creates a place of sanctuary. She is a shepherdess between the two worlds of the spiritual and human, and her skills lie at the point where the emotional and the biological touch each other and interact. She tends the tree of life" (Kitzinger, 2000, p.86).

Midwives that I know, including myself, pray at each birth for Divine guidance. By listening carefully, intuitive messages do indeed come at times of need. Birthing environment needs to be protected not only for the motherbaby but also for the midwife. When the birthing energy is flowing a midwife is able to stay deep within her intuitive self.

Dim lights, maybe some soft music or quietness, warmth, privacy, and lack of distractions are very important for women in labor as this sort of environment takes women out of their thinking brain and puts them in a dreamier state. Giving birth can be very sexual and sensual. During birth, oxytocin is released to bring on contractions and is also the same hormone released to bring on orgasm. (This is not to say you won't release oxytocin during labor if you are not sexually orgasmic.) Endorphins, or natural morphine, are also released, during later labor, and during sexual arousal. This hormone gives you that faraway dreamy feeling. So, during your labor and birth your midwife will make sure that the physical environment is similar to when you make love.

However, after just saying that, some women prefer to have lots of activity and people around them while in labor. There is no right or wrong way to create your environment. Your intuition will guide you in the right direction with respect to what is right for you, and your midwife will work it through with you until your birthing nest is just the way you need it.

Just by observing, a midwife can have a very close idea about how labor is moving along. In early labor the mother begins to spiral inward during contractions. Between contractions the mother may talk, but often her words are questioning as she integrates how her body feels. Her eyes begin to gaze, rather than to look straight at people. She is preparing for her rational mind to quiet down as her intuitive, instinctual self surfaces. She may want to move during, or in-between, contractions, or she may like to just be quietly in one place.

Sometimes birthing energy moves forward quickly. This may catch a mother off guard. The midwife can then offer a steady voice and touch to calm the frantic mother. Soon enough the mother will learn how to face this stronger energy and the midwife can then go back to observer and guardian rather than active participant.

There are many signs in the laboring mother's body that a midwife watches for. These signs indicate that the birthing energy is building. As described before, the mother will go inward as contractions build in intensity, and usually, become longer and closer together. Occasionally, warm-up contractions, leading into early labor, are the same in length and closeness as stronger contractions. What's most important is that the intensity increases. Sometimes women will labor in a waltz pattern of one strong contraction, then two lighter ones, then one strong, two lighter, etc.

During this time of integration it is very important that laboring women are not distracted with questions and endless chatter. The birthing woman's rational mind is now quieted and does not need to be awakened. Any questions or directions aimed at her at this point should be one or two words. "Here's water" and waiting for her body response is all that is needed rather than saying, "Would you like some water? Shall I put ice in it?" The midwife knows to stay aware of what the mother's needs may be. Although midwives are not mind readers, in general it is safe to say that midwives are sensitive to the needs of the mother. However, suggestions from midwives are just those: suggestions. Only the laboring women truly knows what is best for her, but sometimes, an idea or suggestion may be helpful. For instance, the midwife may offer suggestions such as moving to another position, or trying a breathing technique.

The safe passage of the baby is, of course, of utmost importance. The midwife communicates with the baby by listening to the heart tones at least every hour or so during labor and more often while pushing. Heart tones range from 120-160 but are generally lower during pushing.

Some midwives take the blood pressure, pulse, and temperature of the laboring woman to have baseline readings. They also do vaginal checks so they know how far effaced (how thin the cervix is) and how far dilated, or opened, the cervical opening is. Vaginal checks also can give further information on the position of the baby, and how far down into the pelvis the presenting part is. Other midwives feel that vaginal checks, as a ritual for every woman are not necessary, and intrude on the process. They sense that vaginal checks are meddlesome and bring a mother out of her inner space. The information may be discouraging for the laboring woman if she is less far along than she had hoped. The information is somewhat useless as a woman can be dilated to three for hours and then suddenly be nine with a few strong contractions. Or a mother could be dilated to nine and then not have her baby in her arms for several hours later. It is best just to focus on keeping the birthing energy flowing.

There are, however, times when vaginal exams can be useful. If something seems unusual, for instance, the baby's presenting part is in an awkward position, the information gained during a vaginal exam might be useful for giving ideas on what to do next.

Other signs that the midwife looks for are a glazed, glassy appearance of the mother's eyes later in labor. As birthing energy increases so does the rising of the uterus during contractions. You can see that the contractions are stronger. A purple line follows the mother's crack between the buttocks during labor. It is so amazing that the line goes higher with increased dilation.

As the mother's cervix dilates an observant midwife can follow her progress by paying close attention to the color changes of this line. Such a midwife would not need to rely on vaginal checks to chart a laboring woman's progress.

There is a certain smell that emanates from the mother close to birth. The smell is one of hard work, heat and earthiness. When I smell that smell of birth I often will see white light flowing into the laboring mother at the top of her head. The two often are together. Sometimes I see the light through most of a labor. The light definitely is stronger when it is close to birth and becomes more dense about two feet above the head when birth is close.

As birthing energy climaxes there is tension increasing to the point where it seems as though no one in the birthing room, including the midwife, can take any more. Sometimes the midwife feels physical signs, unique to her own body, that birth is imminent. These signs may include sweating, yawning, diarrhea or a need to urinate, or a need to go into a deep trance-like state for a few moments.

And then, there is often a moment of surrender. The energy may change, much like the calm before a thunderstorm. The midwife is prepared for the emergence of this new baby and her/his safe passage. The role of the midwife is to watch, wait, encourage, and listen with an open heart and clear mind. Sometimes she keeps her hands off the whole process and other times she receives the new being into her hands, continuing the momentum of the baby spiraling up into the mother's arms.

Many women like having warm oil applied to their perineum when the baby is crowning. While this may not prevent tears, many women appreciate how the oil feels during perineal stretching. When the baby's head is born the midwife will check to see if the cord is around the baby's neck. Having the cord around the neck is a common occurrence. Usually the cord can be loosened and the baby slides right on through with the next contraction. It can seem as if an eternity has passed between the time when the head is out and the rest of the baby is born. Depending upon what position you are in, the midwife may catch the baby as it slides on out, or perhaps you, the mother, would like to catch your own baby. The baby is placed immediately on the mother's chest and covered with a blanket.

While not disturbing the motherbaby the midwife keeps a very close eye on the transitioning of the baby and for signs of placental separation. Some midwives routinely suction the baby's nose and mouth while others simply let mucous drain out. At this point the midwife must be very alert while not interfering with the bonding of the mother and baby. She must calmly talk as little as possible for the mother is not yet ready to be brought back into her rational mind. Disturbing the mother can lessen her release of oxytocin. It is extremely important that this hormone continue to be secreted at this time because it will stimulate contractions that will release the placenta. The continued release of oxytocin also assures that the uterus will contract well to minimize bleeding.

Oxytocin released after birth is also responsible for bringing on the deep feelings of maternal love for a mother's newly born baby. Michel Odent writes in the *The Farmer and the Obstetrician*, "We know that, in physiological conditions, the mother can reach a high peak of oxytocin, the hormone of love, and also the hormone necessary for the delivery of the placenta. This peak of oxytocin is associated with a high level of prolactin—the motherhood hormone. The association of oxytocin plus prolactin means love for babies" (Odent, 2002, p. 72).

It is the midwife's role to keep the birthing room very warm. So warm, in fact, that anyone else in the room will probably be sweating. A tremendous amount of vital energy has swooshed out of the mother from the birth and the warmth of the room will help her keep her energy in balance. Babies are not able to regulate their temperature for several hours after birth and need warmth to also keep their vital energy within their own bodies.

The placenta is born about twenty minutes after the baby is born. Usually there are about three small gushes of blood that happen when the mother has contractions. The midwife may need to gently bring to the mother's awareness that her placenta is ready to be born. At this point the mother can push out the placenta on her own.

The placenta will be checked to make sure all of the cotyledons, or pieces that were attached to the uterus, are there and that the membranes are intact. The cord will also be checked to be sure that there are three vessels.

Once the placenta is born, the amount of vaginal bleeding is within normal limits, and the baby is dry, warm, and stable, the midwife will observe quietly as the family bonds. The baby is not forced to nurse, but rather is snuggled up to her/his mother's breast. Often nursing is established soon after birth. The midwife will be sure the mother is comfortable before she begins and while she is nursing. Most importantly the midwife must guard this sacred, holy time. This is a time of laying the foundation for a lifetime of relationship.

In the next few hours after birth, while still observing both mother and baby, midwives tidy up the house, do a newborn exam including weighing and measuring the baby, and bring food and drink to the mother. While the mother is up to use the bathroom the bedding is changed, if need be.

Usually after two or three hours the alertness from the adrenaline that both mother and baby received just before and after birth begins to lessen. At this time motherbaby and the new family are ready to snuggle up and have a nap. The midwife then slips quietly out into the world, tired, but satisfied and grateful, that another new life has safely journeyed onto Mother Earth.

~Eight~

Healing the Unexpected

Sometimes life's journeys can take us on a bumpy road. The seasons of pregnancy and motherbaby moon time can give us an emotional roller coaster ride. But then again, a full life includes joy and sorrow; such is the nature of living! Grief, of course, has many levels and the responses vary from person to person. Obviously, the death of a baby, whether from a miscarriage or a stillbirth, is a major loss. There is significant grief when a baby is born who will have life long physical or emotional challenges. There can also be unrecognized grief that may also take even longer to move beyond. There may be intense moments of loss that may be fleeting, or less obvious times of sadness which may last a few days or even longer.

Grief and loss play themselves out in our deepest selves and may come into being for a multitude of reasons. Sometimes mothers feel a sense of loss from no longer being pregnant, or from the change in their relationships and life before baby. It is not uncommon to feel this way and these feelings need to be acknowledged just as a significant loss would be. Creating a new "normal" and adjusting to changes in life takes time. Let yourself have a good cry. "Many people find crying a relief. Rather than being an indication of weakness, tears are often a sign of strength and show that the bereaved person is prepared to work through their [sic] grief. Some people find it difficult to cry, and yearn for tears to release their grief" (www.grieflink.com, 2004).

If there have been complications, an emergency, or unwelcome interventions, there is a whole other aspect of the experience that needs integrating. This integration can take a good bit of time and can be very painful in the process. Mothers may wonder why this happened to them, what they did wrong, how it could be fair, etc. Keeping a journal, talking with a compassionate friend, family member, doula, midwife, or even spending time with a reputable counselor, can help you come to terms with your experience.

Through the years I have heard many stories from mothers who talk about deep sorrow, a feeling of inadequacy, and a loss of trusting themselves at the core of their being. Sometimes they speak of feelings that they could no longer trust their body and that their bodies had let them down. They felt their "womanhood" or "motherhood" was taken away from them—as if they were robbed of their imagined birth experience. Many women felt cheated, or even raped, if their care providers treated them disrespectfully or went against their wishes without explaining why. Here are some stories from women whose experiences were not what they had expected.

I felt as though the cesarean I had was totally unnecessary. It was a Friday afternoon, and admittedly, my labor had been rather pokey throughout the day, and even the night before. My doctor told me that I had until 4:00 p.m. to fully dilate or he would do a cesarean. Well, after being told that, my labor slowed down even more. I now know that I did not feel safe, so therefore my labor was slow. I feel in my gut that if I would have been left alone, or even had a home birth, that my labor would have been very different—it would have been fine.

So any way, I ended up having a c-section at 5:30. At the time I had been convinced that it was the right thing to do even though neither my baby nor I were in any distress. I didn't see my baby until ten o'clock that night; five hours after he was born. The first time I saw him I felt numb. I didn't care if I held him or not. As far as I was concerned somebody else could take care of him. I didn't even want to. It was as if my body thought I never was pregnant or that he was dead or something. My brain was trying to make the rest of me love him but I didn't feel the way I thought I would feel. I did not have these feelings with my next two children who were born naturally. I so totally bonded with them. I have felt guilty about how I have felt about my first child. I never really felt for him as I have the other two children. Of course, I took care of him physically, but I never felt an emotional connection with him. This birth happened twenty-three years ago and I am still sad about it. The doctor said that the reason for the c-section was "failure to progress." I have felt like a failure, all right, for all of these years.

Take a Deep Breath is a poem written by a young mother a few years after an emotionally traumatic birth experience.

Take a Deep Breath

"Take deep breaths, work really hard, and your baby will
come out,"
Says my three-old-son,
As he curls into fetal position,
And lays with his head against my breast.
His thick hair begins to tickle my chin.
This is one of my favorite games.

I breathe.
I grunt, and I make noises.
My son slowly raises his head up.
As if he is breaking through the thick skin of
My abdomen.
He smiles from ear to ear
And giggles as he says,
"It's me, your baby has just been born."
I laugh and each time, my eyes well up
With joy as I look at him.

He squirms around on my chest,
And I wonder how he got so big,
So heavy,
So strong.

It is fun,
This birthing dance we do together.

When the game ends I feel so
Much better than what I
Experienced
As a young girl
In an Iowa hospital.

No one takes him,
It is not an emergency,

It is a birth.
He is right here,
Next to me.
And I feel alive,
I am awake.
He is connected to me,
The way it was intended.

When we get up we are both revived
And we dance and sing
Away our morning together.

And each time I am further healed.
And I am stronger,
With my intentions.
© Teresa LaMendola, 2004

This story tells us about a transfer to the hospital from a home birth.

I couldn't believe it when my dreams of having a
home birth were shattered. After pushing for
several hours my baby was still high up in my
pelvis and was crooked in my pelvis. I tried
walking up and down the stairs, being in hands
and knees and knee-chest positions, and my
midwife even used a rebozo. [A rebozo is a long
cloth that is put under a mother's bottom while the
mother is lying on her back. The midwife then
holds the ends of the rebozo and rocks the mother.
At times she may give a jerk in hopes of moving

the baby to a more favorable position.] We tried everything! Finally we decided to go to the hospital. I was so scared! When we arrived at the hospital my baby's heart tones went down a bit and the doctor decided to do a cesarean without even giving me a chance to think about it. The baby was fine and I, of course, am grateful about that.

For me, I planned and dreamt about my baby's birth just as I planned and dreamt for my wedding day. I wanted things to be perfect. There was a big part of me that felt angry right at first. At first I was mad at my midwife for not being able to do more. And then I was mad at the hospital staff for what seemed like making decisions about my baby and my body without my consent.

When I tried to talk about my feelings people would say that I should just be happy that everything was ok. Eventually I stopped talking about it, but I still felt angry and sad about the experience.

I helped myself by writing about my anger. After the anger was gone I cried a lot. Then I was mad at my own body for failing me. After a few weeks I was able to accept that I can't control everything in life. I feel at peace with the experience now.

Coping with a loss as in this last story can actually be more complicated when the grief becomes buried deep within a person. A support group or better yet, a friend with good listening skills, may be just the ticket for surfacing buried emotions. Emotions are released when there is someone who just listens without judgement. Any kind of creative process activity such as singing, writing, painting or drawing, dancing, etc. can also help release your sorrow.

When coping with grief it is important to take good care of your physical body. Here are some ideas that are found to be helpful:

- ♥ Continue to eat a rainbow of food every day—Sometimes when grieving or feeling depressed people turn to 'comfort' foods, which, unfortunately, often happen to be 'junk' foods.

- ♥ Cry–Let your tears wash away your sadness.

- ♥ Exercise–Try to make yourself get up and move. Exercising will most likely give you more energy. Exercising also releases the body's endorphins that naturally dull your pain and help you to move through your pain and grief and learn to trust your body again.

♥ Listen to inspiring music to help you remember the beauty of being alive.

♥ Take part in a creative project—creative processes can be transformative.

♥ Journal—allow your feelings to flow.

♥ Get a massage as often as possible to relieve emotional tension.

Of course, there are no guarantees that everything will go as you had hoped and dreamed for. There are risks to birth just as there are risks to living in general. Birth is a metaphor for life. Most of the time life rolls on in a smooth fashion. And then again, there are other times when problems occur and we just can never figure out why. At these times having faith and trust that there is a reason and deeper meaning for everything can help get you through.

It can be easy for mothers to beat themselves up over an unplanned experience, especially right at first. I have heard mothers say, "Well, if I only would have eaten better, or gotten more exercise." Or, "Why is God punishing me?" Sometimes Mothers want to place blame on someone else so they blame the midwife or doctor for doing too much or for not doing enough.

The fact is that sometimes things go wrong and we will never know when, or why, the problem happened. We can pretend we know the answers, or blame another human, or sue another for our misfortune, but the truth is that most often the story that is played out has its own needs and is way beyond our understanding. Also, there are simply never any guarantees that everything will go as you wish. Natural process in all of its beauty can also have harsh realities and, most often, prefers not to be controlled. The best that you can do is to take good care of yourself and let the process unfold, as it will.

In reality, the natural processes through the seasons of pregnancy are stronger than any human control. Some of the most tremendous life lessons that I have seen for families are the lessons of surrendering to the loss of imagined control over the process. That is a hard lesson to learn when much of the culture we live in wants to control nature. Sometimes no matter how hard we try, the process will not go as we wish. Sometimes babies are born with physical or mental handicaps they will have for the rest of their lives. Sometimes babies die;

they simply were not meant to be on this planet at this time.

Gratefully, medical help is there when we truly need it. Fortunately, those times are few and far between. It is important to remember that while technology can be life saving, it cannot always make situations perfect. Sometimes things go wrong no matter what. There are divine forces at work here and the mysteries of life, in all of their perplexity, will provide.

If you find yourself grieving please remember that nothing helps you to heal as well as time and love. Take good care of yourself, cry when you need to, and be embraced in the healing arms of your loved ones. Continue to love yourself and remind yourself that you did the best you could. Even in painful situations you will, like Mother Earth, weather the storm.

Section Two:

Maintaining Health

Through the Seasons

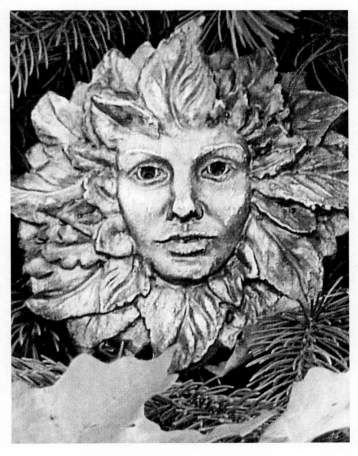

© Janice Marsh-Prelesnik

~Nine~

The Philosophy of Natural Health

Developing your personal natural health care philosophy is a must for living a natural pregnancy. Health is certainly vastly more than the absence of disease. The bottom line principal of natural health is maintaining a flow of balance to your life. In the book *World Medicine*, Tom Monte writes, "Paradox and balance were the basis for all traditional medical systems...health depends upon balancing opposing forces that exist in the body, and in all of life" (Monte, 1993, p.323).

Striving for balance involves several guiding principles towards acquiring natural health. Staying healthy naturally is a way of life: a way of being. Being healthy means feeling balanced, contented, and peaceful. These feelings are essential to the ultimate creation of growing and birthing a baby. Of course breathing fresh air, eating wholesome foods, drinking lots of water, enjoying the sunshine, getting gentle exercise, and sleeping as much as needed are paramount for a healthy three seasons of pregnancy, giving birth naturally, and the season of motherbaby moon time.

Just as important, however, are being nurtured by family, friends, and care giver, eliminating as much stress as possible from the body/mind, and hearing or reading positive pregnancy/birth/new mothering stories. Also, always remember that your intuition and instincts will guide you towards deep ways of knowing and understanding natural health and natural processes. They are your best teachers!

"The ancients understood that health is not a static state, but a fluid one that is continually adapting to its environment"(Monte, 1993, p.323). Our lives flow from moment to moment. Awareness of this flow requires that we intuitively pay attention to the energetic needs of our body. Especially during the seasons of pregnancy it is important to pay attention to the rhythms of each experience. Sometimes more sleep is required, or more food, or a certain kind of food. Or quiet alone time is needed, instead of attending a gathering. Honor these intuitions and care for them.

As a young mother, one of my favorite authors was Juliette de Bairacli-Levy, who wrote about herbalism and natural living for people and animals. Her classic book, *Natures Children: A Guide to Organic Foods and Herbal Remedies for Children,* is now out of print, but well worth while looking for in your library. The following is one of my favorite quotes from this book.

> The health of every family begins with the mother. She is the tree from which the healthy fruit must come. All primitive peoples recognize this, and there are numerous simple laws which the mother is taught to follow to ensure easy and almost painless childbirth and the production of healthy stalwart infants who sleep well and vigorously drink their mother's milk (de Bairacly-Levi, 1970, p.13).

In our fast paced technological culture it can be tricky to follow the laws of staying healthy in a holistic way. How do we create for ourselves a peaceful environment, leading to balance, when there are so many outer voices screaming for our attention? How can we shut out the negativity of the media and stories we hear?

It is important to guard yourself against as many unpleasant experiences as possible, for the emotions that run through you also run through your baby. So think twice before allowing yourself to be bombarded with horror and violence at the movies or on television, or negativity from reading the paper or watching the news. The mother's heart makes the baby's heart; that is to say that your emotions do enter your baby. A baby is very sensitive to what her/his mother is feeling.

In many earth-based cultures the pregnant woman is guarded from harmful feelings and experiences. Carroll Dunham, an anthropological researcher writes in her book, *Mamatoto*,

> Women in Jamaica have traditionally believed that anything upsetting that the mother sees can upset the baby's development, and such things must therefore be avoided. Ibo women of Nigeria believe that if they're faced with a frightening sight they should put their hands over their navel so the baby won't see. Western medicine now believes that any kind of stress and anxiety during pregnancy can make labour more difficult—as if, the Nyinba say, "The baby is fighting with you" (Dunham, 1986, p.49).

Protect yourself from the negativity of the world by imagining you and your baby inside the nurturing, protective bubble that we talked about earlier. Imagine that any negativity directed towards you bounces off the bubble; sending it right back where it came from. In general, Western thought and mainstream culture are often unaccepting of the desire to move into a natural lifestyle. People are often afraid of what is not within their own personal experience, which makes it hard for them to accept and understand someone else's desires. Their concerns may come across to another as negativity.

Relaxing music can also reduce stress and negativity. Your baby will also enjoy listening to music, however muffled it may be, in utero. Singing lullabies to your baby while pregnant is also a lovely way to calm the external chaos of the world. "It is intuitive that there is a profound interplay of information and emotions involved in this sacred and precious dialogue, [of mother singing to baby]" writes anesthesiologist and member of International Society for Music in Medicine, Fred Schwartz (1997, p.3). "Music alone has been shown to diminish stress-induced increases in stress hormones" (Spintage & Droh, 1987, p.88). Listen to calming and relaxing music, or sing your heart out, and the harmonic choirs will sing with you and your baby.

Another insulator is to surround yourself with women who share your values and desires to be a natural mother. Spend time with those who empower you and understand your way of thinking and being. Listen to their stories. Out of their experiences decide what makes sense for you and absorb those positive words. You mustn't let other women's nightmare stories enter and find a home in any cell of your body. Their words may create fear and insecurity. These are not feelings you need to be taking on! Protect yourself. That energy was someone else's and not the energy you wish to create!

The work of Dr. Masura Emoto clearly shows the impact that words can have on physical matter, specifically water. Using high-speed photography Dr. Emoto has photographed frozen water crystals that have been exposed to loving, kind thoughts. These water crystals were beautifully formed, symmetrical, colorful crystals. In contrast he photographed water crystals that had been exposed to anger and negative thoughts. These photographs show that this water was chaotic, asymmetrical in form and dull colored. He also compared water that had been exposed to different types of music. He once again found that certain types of music formed snowflake like crystals. Loud, angry, rock and roll music created disorder in the water. Think about it. The spoken word and music are vibrations. Our bodies consist of a very high ratio of water to our other tissues. It is no wonder we are so sensitive to thoughts, words, and all the vibrations around us. "Water—" writes Dr. Emoto, "so sensitive to the unique frequencies being emitted by the world—essentially and efficiently mirrors the outside world" (Emoto, 2004, p.43).

During your seasons of pregnancy and motherbaby moon time your senses are heightened seemingly a million times over, and I can't stress enough how important it is to keep yourself safe and protected, calm and serene, so that your intuitive body/mind can collect strength and wisdom. This is the foundation for living naturally and developing a natural health care philosophy.

There is no better teacher than Mother Nature herself for showing you the ways of living naturally. "Mother earth, mother nature—she is the literal womb of life, providing all that we need. Her living soil feeds us; her rocks make our bones, her minerals are in our life's blood" (Starhawk, 2004, p.158). Yes, Mother Nature whispers her secrets to us if we quiet ourselves enough to listen. Spend as much time outdoors as possible observing the rhythms and processes of life. Just as the sprouts will burst forth at the right time, know that you too are a part of the natural cycles of the earth. Your baby will be born at just the right time, and you, the vessel for new life, will give birth when the heavens open up for this new being. "To every thing there is a season and a time to every purpose under heaven" (Ecclesiastes 3:1, King James Bible).

Nature teaches you about some of the deep mysteries of life. Walk barefoot in the grass or the sandy beach, watch the breathtaking beauty of the sunrise and sunset, listen to the birds and insects, walk in the woods, stand in awe at the beauty of the earth. Wonder at how the seasons change. Understand that the tremendous energy going through you during birth is the same sort of power as the force of ocean waves moving towards shore. Know that just as a bird knows how to build its nest, and when to lay its eggs, you too will build your birthing nest. Instinct will tell you when to build and intuition will tell you how.

♥ One of the best ways to experience the depth of the wisdom of the earth is to find your own sacred spot to go to every day. Just sit quietly for a few minutes. Use all of your senses to turn inward and outward. Close your eyes and breath deeply—in through the nose and out through the mouth. Imagine that you are cradled in the womb of the Earth Mother and are protected in her sheltering arms, just as your baby is sheltered in the warmth of your womb. Feel the energy and pulse of your own life. Sit in your sacred spot every day of every season. Feel the heat or cold, feel the gentle breeze or the icy, stinging wind. Whatever season you are in remember that in life there are gentle, pristine moments, and also harsh realities. The extremes of nature are a metaphor for the seasons of your pregnancy. Remember that as each season spirals to the next, so too will your life. Weaving emotions and thoughts, and physical sensations in and out—this is a time for letting you feel deeply all there is to feel.

Gardening is wonderful exercise, which keeps the body and the spirit strong. While stretching, bending, and squatting, you can also experience the oneness of being in nature. Soon you will be rewarded for your hard work with fresh vegetables and fruits to nourish you and your baby, and flowers to delight your eyes and nose. Plant an organic garden and you don't have to worry about harmful chemicals! There are many organic gardening books on the market for you to research. Better yet, find an organic gardener in your community. The gardeners that I know are more than happy to share their love of the green world, especially if you pull a few unwanted plants for them while you are chatting.

I have an engraved rock in my herb garden that reads, "To Cultivate a Garden is to Walk With God." The joy of watching a plant grow, that you planted and nurtured, is satisfying, and is a similar feeling to marveling at the growth of your baby. While you are exercising, gardening brings a sense of inner peace to your entire being. This is also multi-tasking (a skill that is very useful for mothering) at its best!

Walking is also a great way to exercise while pregnant, and with a new baby. Walk in the woods, along the sandy beach, listen to the crunch of leaves in the autumn, and enjoy the twinkling of fresh snow on a sunny winter day. Your baby will enjoy the rhythmic movement while you take in the smells, sights, and sounds. Fresh air will do you both good. Who knows, maybe your baby will even be accustomed to the sounds of nature before she or he is even born. Continue your walks as soon as possible after birth with your baby snuggled close to you. Walk briskly, but also don't forget to "stop and smell the roses." Keep your observation skills alert and marvel at the design of nature.

Are you lucky enough to live near a lake or the ocean? Swimming is especially wonderful in the latter months of pregnancy. While being suspended in water, seemingly weightless, your body can move without feeling stressed. I loved to swim in Lake Michigan while pregnant, especially when the waves were rolling in. I often imagined that the floating feeling of being in the water was what my baby was feeling.

Our bodies were made to move and it is very important to keep moving during pregnancy. Keep yourself physically strong and develop stamina. Yoga and Tai Chi are also strengthening exercises. They build the body, mind, and the breath. You can find a form of exercise that you enjoy which will keep your body limber and stretched.

It is important to listen carefully to the wisdom of your body through the seasons of pregnancy and motherbaby moon time. When the body asks for movement, move. When your intuitive sense says that's enough, stop. Don't push yourself to exhaustion. If you enjoy riding your bike, but feel leery in the latter parts of pregnancy, stop riding. Walk instead. You will know when an exercise is not right for you.

Remember that during pregnancy you are breathing for two. With each breath gather in as much oxygen has you can. Each cell in your body needs oxygen. Watch how a newborn baby breathes. Her/his belly rises with each breath as the diaphragm pushes down to allow the lungs to fully expand. Somewhere in life most people in our culture forget how to breath deeply like babies do. Stress is one factor that keeps us from breathing deeply.

It is interesting that deep breathing can help eliminate stress and put you in a more calm, peaceful state. Practice slow, deep breathing and make it a part of your being for the rest of your life. Think of a balloon inside your belly that fully expands with each breath. Breathe slowly, in through the nose and out through the mouth. Your exhale should be as long, or longer, than your inhale. Make this a habit. It will serve you well during labor.

Sleeping as much as needed is also an integral part of living a natural health style. During the early weeks of pregnancy you will most likely find that you are extremely tired. Follow your body's cues and sleep as much as you need to. This sleep time allows the little placenta to firmly attach to your uterus. It is nature's way of protecting your tiny baby and it allows your body to get used to the enormous changes it is experiencing. Also, your body/mind will have more time to integrate the immense idea that you are now a mother! Don't be surprised if you have vivid, interesting dreams at this time. The miracle of a new life is a lot to process! During the last few weeks of pregnancy it is very important to get as much sleep and rest as needed, as you wouldn't want to enter into the work of labor tired. When the baby is born you will learn to sleep when he or she sleeps.

Don't forget to drink a lot of clean water to bathe every cell of your body. Your body is 80% water and that fluid needs to constantly be replenished. Every morning fill at least two quarts of water and make sure you have emptied them by the end of the day.

Eat whole foods, which are still alive, as close to their natural state as possible. Eat lots of fresh vegetables and fruits, organic when possible. The energy of the green world will enter you. Nutrition is so important that I have devoted the next chapter to it.

Marvel at the great design of yourself, and your baby. As you develop your own natural health care philosophy remember that only you know what is best for you, your baby, and your family. Live well, live happy, live naturally!

~Ten~

Eat a Rainbow Everyday:
Nourishment for Motherbaby

Eat a rainbow of colorful foods every day and you will be well on your way to excellent nourishment for yourself and your baby. It is a rather daunting thought when you realize that your baby is totally dependent on you alone for nutrition throughout the seasons of pregnancy and early nursing. What you eat will have a huge impact on how you feel during your pregnancy, the growth of the placenta, and the future health of your baby. Strive to eat colorful foods, which are organic, and grown near you, as much as possible. Why do I recommend organic foods when they are typically more expensive than conventionally grown food? What does organic farming mean?

Organic farming is an agricultural system that encompasses:

- ♥ Management practices that sustain soil health and fertility
- ♥ The use of natural methods of pest, disease, and weed control
- ♥ High standards of animal welfare

- ♥ Low levels of environmental pollution
- ♥ Enhancement of the landscape, wildlife, and wildlife habitat
- ♥ The prohibition of all genetically engineered food and products (www.soilassociation.org, 2004)

Plants grown organically have more nutrition available to them. Studies carried out by Virginia Worthington, Sc.D., have shown that organically grown fruits and vegetables on the average contain 27 percent more vitamin C, 21 percent more iron, 29 percent more magnesium, 14 percent more phosphorus, and 15 percent fewer nitrates than conventional produce (Worthington, 2003, p. 1).

Organic fruits and vegetables may not be as large as conventionally grown produce that you see in the supermarket. Synthetic fertilizers tend to make plants grow quickly. Although organic produce may be smaller in size, the food is more densely packed with flavor and energy. If you have ever eaten a wild strawberry and compared it to a cultivated strawberry you understand that size is not always the most important aspect of a food. A tiny wild strawberry packs a punch in regards to taste and vibrancy.

Researchers at the University of California recently discovered that organically grown produce is higher in cancer-fighting phenolics (antioxidants plants use to defend themselves) than produce sprayed with pesticides and herbicides (Worthington, 2003). It is as if the plants themselves are stronger if they are allowed to grow organically. That strength enters our body when we eat these foods.

"Studies suggest that chronic low-level exposure to OP (organophosphorus pesticides) may effect neurological functioning, neurodevelopment, and growth in children" (Hood, 2003, p.1). Keep away from those pesticides and herbicides as much as possible for the health and well being of you and your baby. Not too long ago I was the midwife for a family who had recently bought a grape farm. The label on the pesticides that were used for the grapes read, "...do not allow children near area where sprayed for 30 days." The man of this family was very discouraged when reading this, because he moved to the farm so that his children could be out in the fields playing while he worked. He is now in the process of switching to organic methods of grape growing. Who really knows the long-term effects of pesticides and herbicides on the human body?

"The biochemical and energetic nutrients which we digest, absorb, and metabolize from foodstuffs, are the foundation of all cellular activity in the body, including growth, repair, reproduction, resistance to disease, and maintenance. Good nutrition is critically important to every form of life we know (Weed, 1989, p.13).

Here is one more thought about buying food from local, diversified, organic farms. These farmers, like you, are following a path less taken, and believe in the value of studying and following natural process. Let's support one another in the quest for natural living and following the laws of nature. For the momentum of natural living lifestyles to keep growing, we truly all need to support one another!

However, if you have the space, grow your own food. Let the food ripen on the plant for the most nutrient dense, alive food you can find. The plant will send all of its energy and nutrition to the fruit or seeds of its labor. Plants, like you, want nothing more than to grow healthy offspring, and send an immense part of their energy and nutrition to reproduction.

If you don't have any available garden space you can still buy local produce. Many cities have garden space to rent, or consider buying produce from a local diversified farm. Community supported agriculture (CSA) is now becoming common around the world. CSA farms grow the food and each family buys a share of the harvest. Produce can be picked up each week at the farm, or sometimes food shares can be picked up at Farmers' Markets in towns.

In the book *The Earth Path: Grounding Your Spirit in the Rhythms of Nature,* author Starhawk writes,

> When we eat something, we literally take in the minerals and energy of the place where it was grown. In an indigenous culture, almost everything people ate came from the land they lived on. Their bodies were literally made of the same stuff as their land. People downriver or over the hill would have smelled different. Myth and religion reflected this close identity. In Mayan mythology, for example, people were made of corn…To eat, then, was not just to take in a set of chemical nutrients. It was to be in profound relationship with a place—with the energies, elements, climate, and life community of that spot on the earth—to ingest the place and become it (Starhawk, 2004, p. 117).

Give your baby, and yourself, the best nutrition by eating fresh foods, grown near you and as close to their natural state as possible. Wild foods such as dandelion, chickweed, and nettles are free foods that are highly nutritious. Also, choose foods with the highest nutritional value. In general, that means eating foods with lots of color. Remember, virtually everything you put in your mouth will go to your baby.

Nutrition Basics

To maintain health and to grow a healthy baby you need to eat a variety of foods from four main categories, which are: water, proteins, carbohydrates, and fats. Vitamins and minerals are found in these foods. For optimal health it is important to eat these foods in the correct balance.

Water

Every cell in our body is bathed in water. Water is essential for every body process. During pregnancy your blood volume expands by 50 to 60 percent. This necessary expansion can not occur without proper water intake. Water transports wastes out, and brings nutrition and oxygen into cells. Without enough water intake elimination of waste through the urinary and digestive systems is inhibited. Water helps us to regulate our internal temperature by eliminating water through the pores of our integumentary system, or skin. It is absolutely imperative that you drink at least two-three quarts of water per day during pregnancy, and even more when nursing. Remember that not only are you drinking for yourself, but you are also drinking for your baby. So keep your water bottle with you wherever you go!

Proteins

Protein creates and builds new tissue. You need a lot of protein during pregnancy to grow a baby and to repair and maintain your own body. When protein foods are eaten the body breaks the components down into amino acids. There are twenty-two known amino acids. When the body is building new tissue it takes the amino acids it needs and synthesizes them to grow the new tissue. Such wisdom on the body's part!

Proteins from animal origins, such as eggs, dairy, poultry, fish, and meats, have complete amino acids. "Although is is important to consume the full range of amino acids…it is not necessary to get them from meat, fish, poultry, and other complete protein foods. In fact, because of their high fat content—as well as the use of antibiotics and other chemicals in the raising of poultry and cattle—most of those foods should be eaten in moderation" (Balch, 1997, p. 4).

Plant proteins can be combined to make complete proteins, thereby acquiring all of the amino acids needed. For instance, rice and beans do not by themselves have all of the amino acids. However, if you combine them, they do indeed complement one another and contain all of the amino acids. To make a complete protein from plant origins combine at least two of the following foods in each meal: brown rice, beans, wheat, nuts, corn and/or seeds (Balch, 1997, p.4).

Carbohydrates

Carbohydrates are energy sources composed of sugars and starches. They give the body the energy it needs to function. When carbohydrates are eaten they are digested and broken down into simple sugars, or glucose, which are absorbed into the bloodstream. Any extra glucose is converted into glycogen and stored in the body, which leads to an excess of body fat.

Carbohydrates are classified into three groups:

♥ Polysaccharides(complex carbohydrates)—starch, glycogen, cellulose, and fiber. Food sources are potatoes, rice, corn, grains.

- ♥ Monosaccharides(simple carbohydrates)—simple sugars such as glucose, fructose, and galactose. Food sources are honey, fructose (sugar in fruits).

- ♥ Disaccharides(simple carbohydrates)—sugars, sucrose and maltose, formed from two monosaccharides. Food sources are cane or beet sugar.

Complex carbohydrates release sugars into the body slower than simple carbohydrates, therefore giving a more sustained effect of energy. Strive to eat complex carbohydrates and monosaccharides. The vitamins and minerals in fresh fruits and vegetables can not be replaced in a vitamin pill. It is also best to avoid processed sugars (www.diet-and-health.net, 2004).

Fats

We need a small amount of fat in our diets for energy and to support growth. Fats are composed of building blocks called fatty acids. There are three main categories of fatty acids:

- ♥ Saturated fatty acids—mostly found in animal foods, such as meat and dairy products, generally solid at room temperature

♥ Polyunsaturated fatty acids—found in vegetable oils such as corn, sunflower, soybean, and safflower

♥ Monounsaturated fatty acids—found in olive, canola, and peanut oils

Fats provide energy and are a catalyst for the fat-soluble vitamins A, D, E, and K. "Rather than thinking of a `low-fat` diet, think of a `right-fat` diet. Growing babies and moms need fats; they provide special components for many of your developing baby's organs—especially the brain, which is 60 percent fat. In fact, the brain grows more rapidly in the womb than at any other stage of human development" (Sears, 2001, p. 46).

Vitamins

Vitamins from foods are organic nutrients that are needed for growth, repair, and maintenance of the body. Vitamins work hand in hand with enzymes. Enzymes are proteins that are made in the body and are needed to transport vitamins to cells and eliminate wastes from cells. They also play a major role in growth, metabolism, cellular reproduction, and digestion (Frye, 1995, p. 205).

Minerals

Minerals are inorganic compounds that every cell is dependent on for survival. Minerals are needed for balancing body fluids, muscle contraction, formation of bone, teeth and blood, and a healthy nervous system. Minerals depend on balance in the body. If one mineral is lacking the others will not be utilized within the cells.

While researching the literature for this chapter I found conflicting ideas on proper nutrition. Some researchers and dieticians feel that the recommended daily allowance (RDA) of nutrition is low while others feel it is adequate. What I advise the mothers I midwife for is to eat as much of a variety of colorful foods as possible, every day. What does seem clear is that foods that are intensely colored have the most nutrition. "Intensely colored foods, such as tomatoes, peppers, blueberries, and spinach, are packed with antioxidants, including vitamins (such as C and E), carotenoids (such as beta carotene, lycopene), minerals (such as selenium) and polyphenols (in red wine and tea)" (Durbin, 2004, p.1).

There is also a new idea in the nutrition world called food synergy. This is based on the idea that combining colorful foods may have benefits that are much greater than the sum of their parts. Fill your plate with a rainbow of color, and not only is your food a feast for the body, but also for the eyes and soul. This is holistic nutrition!

The focus should be on eating organically grown whole foods, as fresh as possible, with the highest nutritional content. Whole foods that are fresh have molecular structures that the human body has tolerated for thousands and thousands of years. The synthetic nutrients that are replaced in processed foods don't have the same molecular shapes as those that are natural. I think of it like this; many people are allergic to synthetic perfumes, but not essential oils (essences that come directly from plants). This is because the molecules of essential oils fit tightly into the smell receptors of the nose, while synthetic smells, which cannot be exactly replicated in molecular shape, are not able to fit tightly into the smell receptors. The nose sees this as a foreign invader and tries to eliminate it by sneezing it out. Could our digestive systems possibly react to synthetic nutrients as foreign invaders? Could synthetic, processed foods cause allergies?

"When I was young I ate a processed food diet. I did not feel well," commented Lorelei, *"then as a young adult I became involved in food co-ops and I started*

eating whole foods. I felt so much more alive. Food is medicine. If we eat well our bodies will be stronger. I do spend more money on whole foods than I would on processed foods. For my family and me it is worth it. I believe if I spend more money on food I will spend less on health care."

Ruth Ann had this to say about eating whole foods. *"When I eat whole, fresh foods I feel as if the energy of the food is entering my body. I feel more alive when I eat live foods! I feel nourished and energized. I think that processed foods leave people feeling unnourished and with a lack of energy. Then they want more food to try and satisfy their need to be nourished. For me it is worth it to grow my own food or to spend more for organic, whole foods."*

Micronutrients

Let's have a look at micronutrients (vitamins and minerals), how they work in the body, and foods that contain high amounts of nourishment. Also included will be herbs and wild foods, which are some of the most nutrient dense foods there are! Much of the information here has been gleaned from one of my favorite nutrition books, *Prescription for Nutritional Healing,* by James and

Phyllis Balch. This popular book can be found in most libraries, bookstores, and health food stores.

Individual Vitamins

Vitamin A

- ♥ Purpose: Maintains healthy skin, supports vision, works as an antioxidant, enhances immunity
- ♥ Foods: Apricots, asparagus, broccoli, cantaloupe, carrots, fish oils, greens (collards, dandelion, beets, kale, mustard, swiss chard, turnip), spinach, dark green leafy lettuces, papaya, peaches, pumpkin, squash
- ♥ Herbs: Alfalfa, nettles, chickweed, parsley, and red clover (together these herbs make a delicious tea)
- ♥ Note: Massive amounts of Vitamin A can be harmful to the liver. This occurs when supplements are taken. It is best to get this vitamin from foods.

Vitamin B Complex

- ♥ Purpose: In general the B vitamins work together. They work to maintain a healthy nervous system, by supporting proper brain function, reducing anxiety, and helping to avoid or relieve depression. They help us have energy by helping to convert carbohydrates to glucose.

Thiamine (B1)

- ♥ Foods: Whole grains, brown rice, meats, fish and poultry, egg yolks, legumes, nuts
- ♥ Herbs: alfalfa, burdock root, chickweed, fennel seed, nettles, oat straw, parsley, peppermint, red clover, red raspberry leaf, rose hips

Riboflavin (B2)

- ♥ Foods: Cheese, egg yolks, meat, fish and poultry, legumes, spinach
- ♥ Herbs: Alfalfa, burdock root, catnip, chamomile, chickweed, nettles, oat straw, parsley, peppermint, red clover, red raspberry leaves, rose hips

Niacin (B3)

- ♥ Foods: Broccoli, carrots, cheese, corn, flour, dandelion greens, dates, eggs, fish, dairy, peanuts, potatoes, tomatoes, wheat germ, and whole wheat products
- ♥ Herbs: Alfalfa, burdock root, catnip, chamomile, chickweed, fennel seed, licorice, nettle, oat straw, parsley, peppermint, red raspberry leaf, red clover, rose hips

Pantothenic Acid (B5)

- ♥ Foods: Whole grains, wheat germ, legumes, mushrooms, nuts, fresh vegetables, meat, fish, poultry

Pyridoxine (B6)

- ♥ Foods: Carrots, chicken, eggs, fish, meat, peas, spinach, sunflower seeds, walnuts, wheat germ
- ♥ Herbs: Alfalfa, catnip, oat straw

Cyanocobalamin (B12)

- ♥ Foods: Dairy products, seafood, and sea vegetables, soybeans, nutritional yeast
- ♥ Herbs: Alfalfa, bladderwrack, hops

Biotin

- ♥ Foods: Egg yolks, meat, dairy, saltwater fish, soybeans, whole grains, brown rice

Choline

- ♥ Foods: Egg yolk, legumes, meat, milk, soybeans, whole grains, wheat germ

Folic Acid

- ♥ Purpose: Folic acid is so very important during pregnancy. Deficiencies during the first trimester can encourage "deformities such as cleft palate, brain damage, spina bifida, slow development, and poor learning ability in the child. A deficiency has been found in mentally retarded children. Folic Acid should be taken [or better eaten] six weeks before conception. In addition, a deficiency may lead to toxemia [pre-eclampsia], premature birth, afterbirth hemorrhaging, and megaloblastic anemia in both mother and child (Kirschmann, 1996, p.66). The word folic has the same roots as foliage i.e. eat your GREENS every day!

♥ Food: Barley, brown rice, cheese, chicken, dark green leafy vegetables, legumes, lentils, milk, mushrooms, oranges, split peas, salmon, tuna, wheat germ, whole grains

Inositol

♥ Foods: Citrus fruits, dairy, meat, nuts, whole grains, vegetables

Para-Aminobenzoic Acid (PABA)

♥ Foods: Whole grains, mushrooms, spinach, dark green leafy vegetables

Vitamin C

♥ Purpose: Prevention of colds, antioxidant support, tissue growth and repair

♥ Foods: Berries, cherries, citrus fruits, dark green vegetables, green peppers, potatoes, pumpkins, squash, strawberries, tomatoes

♥ Herbs: Alfalfa, burdock, chickweed, dandelion, fennel seed, peppermint, nettle, oat straw, parsley, plantain, red raspberry leaf, red clover, rose hips, violet leaves and flowers

Vitamin D

♥ Purpose: Needed for calcium absorption, required for healthy bones and teeth Fat-soluble vitamin

♥ Foods: Dairy products, fish liver oils, saltwater fish, eggs yolks

♥ Herbs: Alfalfa, dandelion, nettle, parsley

Vitamin E

♥ Purpose: Strengthens smooth muscle and works as an antioxidant

♥ Foods: Cold pressed vegetable oils, dark green leafy vegetables, legumes, nuts, seeds, whole grains

♥ Herbs: Alfalfa, dandelion, nettle, oat straw, red raspberry leaf, rose hips

Vitamin K

♥ Purpose: Needed for formation of blood clots

♥ Foods: Asparagus, broccoli, Brussel sprouts, cabbage, dark green leafy vegetables, egg yolks, whole grains

♥ Herbs: Alfalfa, green tea, nettle, oat straw

Bioflavonoids (Vitamin P)

- ♥ Purpose: Aids absorption of vitamin C
- ♥ Foods: Black currents, buckwheat, citrus fruits (white part underneath skin), peppers
- ♥ Herbs: Elderberries, hawthorn berry, rose hips

Individual Minerals

Boron

- ♥ Purpose: Aids in metabolism of calcium, phosphorus, and magnesium
- ♥ Foods: Apples, carrots, grapes, green leafy vegetables, nuts, pears, grains

Calcium

- ♥ Purpose: Necessary for bones and teeth, muscle contraction, nerve impulses, regulates heart rate
- ♥ Foods: Almonds, dairy foods, dark green leafy vegetables, sardines, seafood, sesame seeds, spinach, and all greens
- ♥ Herbs: Alfalfa, burdock root, chickweed, dandelion, fennel seed, nettle, oat straw, parsley, peppermint, plantain, red raspberry leaves, red clover, rose hips, violet leaves and flowers

Chromium

- ♥ Purpose: Aids in metabolism of glucose and synthesis of protein and fats
- ♥ Foods: Brown rice, cheese, meat, potatoes, whole grains
- ♥ Herbs: Catnip, licorice, nettle, oat straw, red clover

Copper

- ♥ Purpose: Helps in formation of bone, hemoglobin, and red blood cells
- ♥ Foods: Almonds, avocados, barley, beans, beets, broccoli, seafood, nuts, oats, green leafy vegetables

Germanium

- ♥ Purpose: Carries oxygen to cells
- ♥ Foods: Garlic, shiitake mushrooms, onions
- ♥ Herbs: Aloe vera, comfrey, ginseng

Iodine

- ♥ Purpose: Thyroid gland depends on iodine for good health, helps to metabolize fat
- ♥ Foods: Sea salt, iodized salt, seafood, saltwater fish
- ♥ Herbs: Bladderwack, kelp

Iron

- ♥ Purpose: Essential for hemoglobin formation. Hemoglobin carries oxygen to our cells
- ♥ Foods: Almonds, eggs, fish and meat, green leafy vegetables, whole grains
- ♥ Herbs: Alfalfa, burdock root, catnip, chickweed, dandelion, nettle, oat straw, parsley, peppermint, plantain, red raspberry leaf, rose hips, yellow dock

Magnesium

- ♥ Purpose: Supports calcium and potassium assimilation.
- ♥ Foods: Dairy foods, fish, meat, seafood, fruits, green leafy vegetables
- ♥ Herbs: Alfalfa, bladderwrack, catnip, chickweed, dandelion, nettle, oat straw, parsley, peppermint, red raspberry leaf, red clover

Manganese

- ♥ Purpose: Essential for protein and fat metabolism
- ♥ Foods: Egg yolks, green leafy vegetables, legumes, nuts

Molybdenum

- ♥ Purpose: Promotes normal cell functions
- ♥ Foods: Beans, grains, legumes, peas, dark green leafy vegetables

Phosphorus

- ♥ Purpose: Bone and tooth formation
- ♥ Foods: Asparagus, wheat bran, corn, dairy products, eggs, fish fruit legumes, nuts, sunflower, sesame, pumpkin seeds, meats, and poultry

Potassium

- ♥ Purpose: Needed for nervous system, muscle contraction, and regular heartbeat
- ♥ Foods: Bananas, brown rice, dairy foods, fish, fruit, legumes, poultry and meat, vegetables, whole grains
- ♥ Herbs: Catnip, nettle, plantain, red clover

Selenium

- ♥ Purpose: Antioxidant of lipids, aids in development of antibodies
- ♥ Foods: Seafood, whole grains, sesame seeds
- ♥ Herbs: Alfalfa, catnip, chickweed, fennel seed, hawthorn berry, nettle, oat straw, parsley, peppermint, raspberry leaf, rose hips

Silicon

- ♥ Purpose: Assists in formation of collagen and connective tissue growth
- ♥ Foods: Beets, brown rice, bell peppers, soybeans, leafy green vegetables, whole grains

♥ Herbs: Alfalfa, horsetail

Sodium

♥ Purpose: Needed for maintaining water balance

♥ Foods: Found in almost all foods and herbs

Sulfur

♥ Purpose: Protects cells by making them slightly acidic

♥ Foods: Brussel sprouts, beans, cabbage, eggs, fish, kale, meats, onions, soybeans, wheat germ

♥ Herbs: Horsetail

Vanadium

♥ Purpose: Needed for cellular metabolism and for teeth and bone formation

♥ Foods: Fish, olives, meat, radishes, green peas, vegetable oils, whole grains

♥ Herbs: Dill

Zinc

♥ Purpose: Promotes healthy immune system, needed for reproductive organ health, and health of oil glands

♥ Foods: Egg yolk, fish, legumes, lima beans, meats, mushrooms, poultry, pumpkin seeds, seafood, soybeans, sunflower seeds, whole grains

♥ Herbs: Alfalfa, burdock root, chickweed, dandelion, nettle, parsley, rose hips

To be sure you are eating foods that encompass the entire list of nutrients write down all of foods that you eat throughout a day. Then go through the list of nutrients and make sure that you have eaten a food listed for each vitamin and mineral.

Cait Johnson, writes in her delightful cookbook, *Cooking Like a Goddess; Bringing Seasonal Magic Into the Kitchen,*

> How we eat—our frame of mind and heart—may be just as important as what we eat. We can all name relatives or friends who drink like fish, smoke, eat terrible things, and are eighty years old and still going strong. Likewise, many of us are busy doing all the "right things"—fretting over proper food combinations, cutting out anything remotely "bad" or dangerous (no caffeine, no alcohol), agonizing over every gram of fat, and all the rest of it—and we're not exactly glowing with health. Perhaps the key is to relax, connect with the Earth and the food it gives us, and live joyously...And although there are no guarantees that joyful and connected living will prolong your

life, it will certainly make life a pleasure while you live it (Johnson, 1997, p. 2).

Make meal times a celebration, and don't forget to give thanks to the Mother Earth for providing a rainbow of food for you and your baby!

~Eleven~

Philosophy of Natural Remedies for the Seasons of Pregnancy

Most of the time the body maintains homeostasis—or the ability to keep in balance. Natural forces work within us to help maintain homeostasis. The human body, as well as all organic matter, has the ability to heal and revitalize itself. Consider the impressive miracles of the rejuvenation of the human body.

Every day our blood travels 168 million miles. That's 6,720 times around the earth's globe. We have enough carbon for 9,000 lead pencils and sufficient calcium to completely whitewash a chicken coop. Every five days, our whole intestinal lining is renewed. Every eleven days, our respiratory lining is replenished. Every fifteen days, all our white corpuscles are replaced: it takes 120 days for the red corpuscles. Every six months, we have a new bloodstream. Every eleven months, we have a new cell structure, and we get a new set of bones every two years. An entirely new body is recreated every seven years. Without considering any aspect other than our physical, we are splendid creatures (Pickering, 1998, p.1).

We are indeed splendid creatures. The body has such an enormous capacity to rejuvenate itself. There are times of stress and imbalance, however, when we can aid the rejuvenation and the healing processes with the use of natural remedies. The modalities that I most often use for my family, and myself, and suggest to the families I midwife for, are staying emotionally healthy, and using herbs, massage, aromatherapy, and hydrotherapy to assist with supporting and maintaining health. The healing plants of nature, the balancing nature of water, and the power of touch can nourish and eliminate, or at least greatly lessen, the stresses of life. Stress can be from physical causes, i.e. not eating well, not getting enough rest or exercise, or not drinking enough water, or can be caused by emotional imbalances.

Christiane Northrup, M.D. writes, "Many illnesses are quite simply the end result of emotions that have been stuffed, unacknowledged, and unexperienced, for years" (Northrup, 1993, p.55). Emotional stress will find a home in the spirit/body/mind if we are not able to work it out. Emotional stress can include fear, frustration, anger, sadness, anticipation, grief; in short any feeling that brings on an uneasiness. These stresses become embodied and have an affinity for special areas of the body. When in the body these emotions are heavy and create dark clouds in the area where they are finding their hopefully, temporary home. We all know how heavy and painful they feel. Hence phrases like "I'm carrying the world on my shoulder," or "I feel like I was kicked in the stomach." In my body, frustration shows up as tension and pain in my shoulders and neck. Deep breathing, having a massage, and doing tai chi, are ways that assist my body in eliminating frustration.

On the flip side, too much excitement or joy can also lead to stress. Have you ever been so excited about something that you didn't sleep well and then weren't able to enjoy the next day because you were so tired?

Strive for balance in life by discovering your own healthy coping mechanisms for dealing with stress. Thoughts and emotions do have a chemical makeup, called neuropeptides (Pert, 1993), and can alter your physiology. In *Molecules of Emotion*, Candace Pert writes, "Physiology and emotions are inseparable. I believe that happiness is our natural state, that bliss is hardwired. Only when our systems get blocked, shut down, and disarrayed do we experience the mood disorders that add up to unhappiness in the extreme" (Pert, 1993, p. 265).

While recognizing that you can not eliminate your range of emotions you can, however, teach yourself to neutralize extreme emotions. Acknowledge and rationalize extreme feelings and they will begin to dissipate. How can you do this? If you have allowed another person to upset you, try to see his/her point of view. Forgive this person. Let it go. Is the situation really that important that you will allow yourself to be hurt over it?

These words of wisdom written by Dr. Emoto in *The Hidden Messages of Water* are a great source of encouragement for how to free our souls from extreme emotions.

> Based on the principles of vibration, the answer is very clear. All we need to do is emit the emotion that is opposite to the negative emotion. By combining two opposite waves, the negative emotion disappears... For every negative emotion, there is an exactly opposite positive emotion. The following list contains emotions that create opposing frequencies:

Hate	Gratitude
Anger	Kindness
Fear	Courage
Anxiety	Peace of mind
Pressure	Presence of mind

(Emoto, 2004, p.73).

If you are fearful, find the deep issue of where your fear lies. Delve into it and replace that fear with trust that everything will be ok. Deep breathing, exercise, praying, or meditating are all ways to eliminate stress. Have a good cry. Tears take on a different chemical makeup each time you cry. Do tears help to eliminate negative emotions? I believe so. Throughout most of my life I cried often. A few years ago I decided I would teach myself to "toughen up." Was that ever a mistake! I'm a sensitive person by nature (as we all are), and without tears emotions did find a home within my body. Don't hold back tears. A friend recently told me about a sign she saw which read, "There can be no rainbows in the soul without tears in the eyes." Crying does a body good!

Take on the attitude that life is wonderful and natural process does provide for us. Life is a journey, a grand adventure! Don't allow our fear-based, competitive culture to permeate your being.

Become aware of where you body holds physical stress. The best way I know of to learn where your body is holding tension is to receive a relaxation massage. Pay attention to sensitive tender areas. Why are certain areas sore? Search internally for the answer and think about ways to prevent that tension from continuing. After your massage be aware of what you are experiencing when tension starts to enter your body. Simple things such as carrying a heavy purse over your shoulder can tighten muscles. Carrying a baby on one side can leave you lopsided. Switch sides and stretch out often. Sitting too long can cause tension. Get up and move. Not verbalizing what you want to say can cause a stiff and sore neck. As always the key is balance. Is your tension caused by physical or emotional stress? One of my massage instructors told her students, "You can't take care of anyone else if you don't take care of yourself. Make this your mantra." How true that statement is. Stress, both emotional and physical, is a part of life. But, you can choose whether or not you are going to let it consume you. You are your best healer.

What situations bring stress to you and where are those stresses stored in your body/mind? Take care of it now. Learn to immediately recognize when stress is entering you and strive to deal with it in the moment. Then when your baby grows you can teach your child, by your example, ways to cope with stress. This is one of the greatest gifts you can give to your child.

Ideally, it would be wonderful if we could eliminate as much stress as possible in our daily lives before it could find a home in our bodies. Sometimes this isn't possible, and we need to ask for outside assistance. There are times when nourishment and nurturing are in order. Other times more specific remedies are needed to aid the body in its healing process.

Before we look at specific remedies let's first discuss the philosophies of each of the healing modalities we will be exploring. It is important to understand how the remedies work.

Herbs

Herbs are often my first choice for a natural remedy. I love the green world of herbs and, yes, I even love "weeds." Healing for me begins when I am sitting and working in my medicinal herb garden. My senses overflow with smells, colors, shapes of leaves and stems, the sound of the bees and hummingbirds, the sun and the breeze. "Discovering that our medicine begins in the village—in the fields and woods that surround us, to be precise—is empowering. So many of the good things in this life are simply intended as everyday blessings" (Phillips, 2001, p.xii,). Just being in that garden brings on a deep sense of relaxation and love.

As much as possible get to know the herbs that you wish to use for healing. Just learn a few at a time and learn the plants that live near you, in your bioregion. A few common plants to start with, growing throughout much of North America, are dandelion, catnip, yarrow, plantain, and chickweed. There are many identification books available. Look in your yard, or at the park, and find the most common weeds growing there. After identifying that the herb you are studying is safe for consumption, and assuming it has not been chemically sprayed, sit quietly and hold a stem or root of a fresh herb. Do you feel the plant's life force? What do you smell? Then taste it. Chew it really well. What does it taste like? Does it tingle in your mouth? Is it bitter? Come to know the herb's life cycle, the energies of the plants and marvel at their beauty. Observe the plant's life cycle. Keep a notebook with you and draw the plant at different stages of its growing season. Study the properties of the plants. How does each one work in your body?

In our culture herbs are often used similar to Western medicines, i.e. take the pill to eliminate symptoms. Please don't take on that attitude. It does not do the plants justice. Think of the herbs as nourishers and allies (Weed, 1986) in aiding the body in its own healing process cells.

> The Wise Woman tradition sees everything as nourishment. Nourishment insures life. Nourishment is the great grounding root and green leaf of the Wise Woman tradition. All health occurs through nourishment... Cell by cell, you replace yourself. Thought by thought, you create yourself. Dream by dream, you envision the universe. You create a million new cells every second: impressionable, vulnerable cells. From what do you create them? With what do you imprint them? (Weed, 1986, p.14).

As a natural mother your goal is not to mask symptoms, but to feel deeply and listen to your body/mind and what its needs are. What message is your deep self sharing? Many herbs, including the common "weeds" are full of nourishment. When you make yourself a cup of tea you not only receive the vitamins and minerals of the plant you also are drinking the energy or life force of the plant. The beauty of herbal infusions, or teas, is that you must slow down to make the tea, and sit and relax when you drink it. That is holistic, natural health care at its best!

When problems arise that need further care, herbs can aid the body's innate healing process. For instance, during pregnancy, if you are unfortunate enough to come down with a cold, peppermint facial steams can help to relieve congestion. You can also drink peppermint tea. The idea is not to dry up mucous. Instead you want to make it more watery. Keeping mucous watery enables the body to continue its elimination process going without getting more congested.

In natural healing the object is to allow the body to go through its healing process. This is contrary to Western thought. If you stop symptoms the problem will be sent deeper into the body. Best to let nature take its course, even though it may not always be comfortable. As a natural mother you don't want to take on the Western attitude that life needs to made as easy as possible. The Western way says "Don't feel. Always be comfortable. Get rid of sickness as soon as possible." Fear of pain that is so prevalent in our society keeps people from living fully and deeply. Natural mothers recognize distress, whether it is physical or emotional, as a time to step back and really check in with what is happening in life. Perhaps you need to slow down and take time to "smell the roses", or maybe a baby with the sniffles needs to just sit and be rocked in his/her mother's arms. Of course, I never liked it when my babies were sick, but I fondly remember the loving bond of holding them, sometimes hour after hour, when they didn't feel well. The best healer in the world is mother's love.

"Some of my best memories as a mother with small children were gathering herbs throughout the summer with my children to dry for the winter months," says Ruth Anne. *"Now that my children are young adults they are continuing the herbal legacy of their childhood. Herbs are their first choice when they need further assistance during the healing process."*

Touch Therapies

The healing power of touch is also a readily available natural healing remedy. The idea is to remind the spirit/body/mind to relax so that it can more easily do its work in maintaining balance. There are many types of massage available. They all strive to meet the same goal of relaxation and integrating the whole person.

Touch is as essential to our health as the air we breathe and the food we eat. Of all the senses, touch is the only one we cannot live without. People born without sight or hearing learn to compensate for the absent sense... Without experiencing touch, however, a person may literally perish (Sullivan, 1998, p.17).

A gentle human touch sends love into every cell of the body. The therapeutic effects of massage are enormous. Massage decreases or eliminates muscle pain, increases circulation, decreases anxiety, improves circulation of lymph, and encourages a sense of well being. Endorphins, our body's natural morphine, are increased during massage. During pregnancy, massage can reduce nausea and assist the body in adjusting to the physical changes. The greatest massage I ever received was a few days after my last baby was born. I was the lucky recipient of a one and a half-hour, two-person massage. Aaaaaah! Do yourself a favor and find a massage therapist who knows pregnancy massage, and get a massage, at the very minimum, once a month while pregnant.

There are so many types of massage therapies that it can be a bit confusing to sort through them. Let's have a look at some of the most common. Swedish massage uses kneading, rubbing, light smooth touch, and works on the superficial muscle layers. This is the most common type of massage. Swedish massage warms the muscles as it works out tension.

Foot Reflexology is an ancient therapy that works on the premise that every part of the body is connected or reflexes to a point in the feet. For instance, the toes reflex the head, the balls of the feet reflex the chest and shoulders, the arch area with the abdomen, and the heels with the pelvis and hip area. By stimulating tender areas of the foot, with the thumbs, fingers, or palms, tension is released and sends a free flow of energy to the corresponding body part. I often have shoulder pain and when I do the shoulder point on the same side foot is also sore. One does not need to have formal schooling to give a good foot massage. Have your partner or friend gently massage out sore spots on the feet. If you are retaining fluid in your feet massage up towards the head and at least some of the fluid will move on up too.

Deep muscle therapy is a general term for many specific types of deep tissue work such as Trigger Point Therapy, Rolfing, sports massage, and many others. These types of massage are what you may want to receive if you have specific problem areas such as chronic pain, old injuries, or structural, misalignment problems. As tension releases deep tissue work can be intense and may be painful while the therapist works.

Acupressure is similar to acupuncture but uses touch instead of needles on specific points of the body. There are more than 2,000 acupressure points in the body. In practice, however, a typical acupuncturist's repertoire would be 150 points (Kaptchuk, 1983, p. 5). These points connect to meridians, or channels of energy, that run vertically through the body. Each point corresponds to specific areas of the body. If a meridian is congested, chi, or life force, is unable to run smoothly through the meridian. This congestion brings on pain. When a congested point is held, with the finger or thumb, the congestion is relieved and energy can once again run through the body. Pain and tenderness are then relieved. There are twelve main meridians and eight lesser-known ones.

Energy Therapies

Polarity, and Therapuetic Touch work on a vibrational level. Our little energy packets of protons and neutrons, are busily at work inside every cell in our bodies. The energy becomes chaotic, and instead of flowing smoothly, the protons and neutrons bump into each other and rumble around. This creates pressure in the body, which causes pain and a general feeling of uneasiness. Energy work strives to line up the molecules so that energy is once again flowing smoothly.

An analogy of this is to consider a water hose with a kink in it. When the water is turned on, but unable to move through the hose because of the kink, pressure builds up. The water molecules are still moving, but instead of moving smoothly through the hose, the front ones get backed up and push into the behind ones. The energy becomes chaotic. Release that kink, and whoosh, the energy once again flows. It is like that in our body. Tension, whether physical or emotional, can back up the free flow of energy in our bodies.

When your body/mind is calm and peaceful, your energy is available to freely move through you. It is especially important that you understand this concept during your labor, which is a time when enormous elemental birthing energy is moving throughout your body. This is what moves your baby down and out. If you are tense, and your energy pathways are congested, it can be a struggle for elemental birthing energy to be free flowing.

Mothers are natural energy healers. When a mother kisses an "owie" or puts her hands over a scraped knee she is doing energy work. It's as if love goes through her hands and soothes pain. Just gently and lovingly put your hands where the pain is. You don't even have to touch the skin. You can hold your hands one to two inches above the body and have the similar effect. Hold your hands on or over the sore spot and keep them there until you intuitively feel the energy calm. You may feel heat or a tingly sensation in your hands. Let your hands be your guide. Remember that massage and energy work are intuitive arts.

Aromatherapy

The healing modality of aromatherapy uses essential oils, which are extracts of various parts of the plants. The healing agents of the oils live in the aroma. The smell enters the olfactory membrane, or nose, and journeys to the limbic system where there is an immediate response. The limbic brain is the primitive part of our brain that moderates our emotions, moods, memories, and instincts.

Odor stimuli in the limbic system or olfactory brain release neurotransmitters—among them encephaline, endorphins, serotonin, and noradrenaline. Encephaline reduces pain, produces pleasant, euphoric sensations, and creates a feeling of well-being. Endorphins also reduce pain, stimulate sexual feelings, and produce a sense of wellbeing. Serotonin helps you relax and feel calm. And noradrenealine acts as a stimulant that helps keep you awake (Fischer-Rizzi, 1990, p.27).

The healing properties of the oils also enter the lungs and are absorbed into the blood. The skin will also absorb aromas and then the circulatory system picks up the molecules of aroma. The diffused oil is then transported throughout the body. Each type of oil has a system affinity, meaning that it reacts with certain areas of the body. For instance, the molecules of the aroma of chamomile work well on the digestive system.

Essential oils are powerful. Only one or two drops are needed for a therapeutic effect. Mix them with carrier oil, perhaps olive or sweet almond, and then rub the oil on the skin. Essential oils are eliminated through the lungs during exhalation, the skin, or through the urine. So don't be surprised if you rub cooling peppermint oil on your feet and then smell it in your urine a few hours later.

Hydrotherapy

The last natural healing remedy that we will focus on is hydrotherapy. The use of water for healing may seem quaint, but the simple use of good old water can be powerful. By alternating hot and cold applications of water the body's innate healing system can be stimulated. Congestion of the circulatory and energetic system is relieved. Water can also carry the vital energy and nutrition of herbs and essential oils. Soaking your swollen, pregnant feet in a cold basin of water with a few drops of peppermint essential oil is an example of hydrotherapy, as is sitting in a postpartum sitz bath of healing herbs to help heal your hard working bottom.

Alternating hot and cold compresses can also relieve muscle tension. The general principle of hot and cold applications is to stimulate circulation. Hot is defined as 98-104° (anything hotter is considered dangerous) and cold is defined as 55-65° (Chaitow, 1999, p.10). Hot water opens up blood vessels and cold closes and strengthens vessels, and prevents congestion and stagnation from the hot. In general, cold follows hot applications. Towels can be saturated with water and then wrung out.

Hydrotherapy can also be used to induce fevers by wrapping the person first in hot towels and then in a blanket. You wouldn't want to induce a fever during pregnancy, however, since your baby would also experience the heat.

Each mother must study and embrace natural healing remedies that resonate for her. Lorelei, a natural mother of two, massage therapist, and yoga instructor says,

> *"We use herbal remedies, homeopathy, chiropractic, and massage. My boys generally are healthy; they don't get sick a lot. If I see that they are coming down with something I give them tea, have them adjusted, and I give them massage. I check in with their stress level. For myself, I get adjusted, or get a massage, but mostly I do yoga to maintain health. Yoga is the key for me feeling well. I think when the spine is in alignment everything just flows. Yoga has helped me a lot."*

She goes on to say, *"I think that doctors look in books when they need to know something. And we can do the same thing. We know our children well enough that we can understand their rhythms. We can understand their needs better than a stranger*

> *can. We understand the whole person; we know the whole child."*

Linda, whose partner is a chiropractor says,

> *"We always feel chiropractic would keep our body running the way it is intended to. It keeps the nerves free to do their job. I often was adjusted during my pregnancies. I, of course, avoid things that are harmful. Like synthetic foods, or processed food. It is important to eat foods close to the natural state. We also drink water as our main drink. We use natural vitamins. We have raised seven kids without ever giving them antibiotics. Only one kid ever had an ear infection. We put garlic oil in her ear. It smelled bad but it really seemed to work."*

These are just a few of the many natural-healing modalities available. There are many resources and books to learn from. Of course, there are many other modalities such as homeopathy, Ayurvedic medicine, flower remedies, and others to choose from. Study them and explore modalities that make the most sense for you. Just remember that the aim of natural remedies is to aid the body's innate healing ability, to nourish, and to assist the body in maintaining a calm, relaxed state. Never forget that the greatest healer of all is love!

~Twelve~

Natural Remedies for the Discomforts of Pregnancy

There may be times during the seasons of your pregnancy when your body needs some tender loving care while attempting to remain balanced. Strive for prevention of these discomforts through exercising, eating a rainbow of highly nutritious foods every day, eliminating stress as much as possible, drinking at least two quarts of fluids a day, sleeping and resting as much as needed, and enjoying fresh air and sunshine. All of these should be integrated into your daily routine.

The following remedies may be of assistance to you when prevention isn't enough and your body needs some extra attention. In this chapter we will focus on herbs, essential oils, massage, and nutrition as ways to help alleviate the discomforts and common illnesses that you may encounter during pregnancy.

How can you tell that an imbalance is coming on? Pay attention to how you are feeling at the very beginning of an illness or discomfort. Many times the uneasiness can be avoided if measures are taken at the onset. Ask yourself, "Do I need more rest? Am I emotionally or spiritually stressed? Have I been eating well? Do I need more exercise?" If you answer yes to any of these questions turn the situation around by taking care of the issue at hand. Listen carefully and holistically to the whispers of your entire self. The whispers will soon become shouting and screaming messages if you don't deal with the whispers early on.

Remember that our purpose is not to simply eliminate symptoms. The idea is to assist the body in its healing process. Think through the stages of an illness or discomfort. A backache often occurs simply from staying in one position too long. Pay attention to body cues and get up to move and stretch before muscles become contracted. Contracted muscles cause pain and can move bones out of alignment.

When you feel a scratchy or sore throat coming on one solution is to gargle with some Echinacea root tincture, drink some Echinacea tea, eat foods rich in vitamin C, and have a rest. While resting, send all of the healing energy and love you have to yourself.

To keep healing energy flowing give yourself, or find someone else, to give you a gentle head massage. Use the fingertips and with circular motions spiral out congestion. Pay close attention to tender spots on the scalp, neck and face. Spend more time gently rubbing the congested energy, until it disperses. This massage technique is also wonderful for headaches.

Experience is the best teacher. These remedies that I offer to you are ones that I have used myself and they are what I have suggested to others as their midwife. All of these remedies are safe to use throughout your seasons of your pregnancy and motherbaby moon time.

Of course, there are many other natural remedies to choose from. Many remedies that you could purchase at a health food store are very expensive. The remedies I offer you are the most cost effective; however, they do require more planning and preparation. Herbs mentioned can be used dry or in the fresh form. All of the herbs suggested grow in northern temperate regions. Most of the herbs are easily found along the wayside at the edge of the woods and probably even in your backyard!

Cultivate an attitude of gratitude for all plants that choose to grow near roads. Their ability to clear the air of auto exhaust is amazing. Thank them for what they do but never incorporate them into your remedies and tonics. Follow your intuition, personal experiences, and pocketbook as you discover the remedies that work best for you.

Preparing Herbs

With a little practice it is simple to prepare herbs for use. It is empowering and a joy to make herbal remedies for yourself, your family, and friends. You might be asking, "How will I ever know if my herbal preparations are the right strength?" This takes experimentation and practice. Purchase the preparation from a company and then experiment until your preparation smells and tastes like the bought preparation. Gradually your confidence will grow. Use all of your senses and intuition to guide you. And remember, these herbs have been used throughout time. You are simply remembering what your grandmothers knew. In the *Village Herbalist,* Nancy Phillips writes,

> The ultimate way to test for potency, used in big labs and small kitchens alike, is the *organoleptic method.* Sounds official, doesn't it? Nevertheless, herbalists have been using this test to determine the quality of herbs for eons. The perception of our senses discerns the quality of a particular herb. We use our eye to observe the color and overall details of the plant material. A well-dried herb will retain the Green vibrancy of the fresh plant (Phillips, 2001, p.221-222).

Infusions

Making an herbal infusion is simply preparing a cup of tea. Healing properties of leaves, either fresh or dried, are transported out of the herb and into water when steeped. Use a glass or stainless steel container. First boil the water, turn off heat, add herbs, and then steep for a few minutes. For the greatest amount of healing properties to transfer be sure to steep for several minutes. The taste may be quite strong. Make sure to cover your pot while steeping the herbs to retain the aroma, also called volatile oils. (Remember that babies, and those with more delicate constitutions, will need a weaker brew.) Strain the herbs from the water. Make infusions by the cup or brew a quart jar of herbal tea and sip throughout the day. Infusions will last a day or two in the refrigerator.

Solar Infusions

You can also make sun teas, also called solar infusions. Place the herbs in a jar with a tight fitting lid and leave in the sunshine for a few hours. Solar infusions tend to not bring out bitter flavors. Try making a peppermint infusion this way. It tastes like candy!

Decoctions

Decoctions are made from roots and fibrous herbs. The herb is boiled in the water. Hard and fibrous roots have strong cell walls that will open and let the healing powers escape under intense heat. Boil for a longer period of time than you would steep an infusion: maybe 5-15 minutes. If you are making a brew that has roots and leaves make your decoction first and then infuse the leaves for the last few minutes. With infusions and decoctions, the longer you leave the herbs in the water the stronger the taste will be. Experiment with the process.

Sitz Bath

For a sitz bath or tub bath simply boil all of the plant material together for 20-30 minutes. Strain, and then add to bath. For a sitz bath make sure the healing herbs are not too hot when placed in the tub!

Infused Oils

Infused oils can be used as massage oils, or as a base for salves. To make an infused oil place herbs in a glass jar and then fill the jar again with a vegetable oil. Olive oil is commonly used, although sweet almond oil is also a good choice. It is recommended to use dried herbs in your oil infusions. The water in fresh plants will often turn the oil infusion moldy. Set the oil in the sunshine and let set for 2-3 weeks. More time will be needed if the days are cloudy and cool. You can also make infused oil by using a crock-pot. Cover the herbs with oil and place on low heat for a few hours. Cool the mixture before straining.

To strain put a piece of gauze or linen cloth in a colander. Place the colander on top of a pot. Pour contents into the colander. When most of the oil has dripped through squeeze the cloth with all of your might to extract every last drop of the precious oil.

Salves

To make a salve, add 1/4 cup of grated beeswax to each cup of the warmed, infused oil. Depending on what your preference you could also use cocoa butter, shea butter, or lanolin. Heat slowly and once all of the ingredients are melted together, carefully pour the mixture into jars. Don't move the jars while the mixture is cooling.

Tinctures

Tinctures are potent, concentrated liquid extracts. The folk-way to make a tincture is to fill a jar with the herb, either fresh or dried, and finely chopped, and fill the jar again with a solvent. Most solvents are alcohol, usually vodka, but vinegar and glycerin can also be used.

If you use vinegar be sure to warm it a bit before adding to the plant material as the warmth will initially draw out the essence of the plant. I use inexpensive vodka. Vinegar tinctures are not as potent as alcohol ones. If you use glycerin as your solvent be sure to dilute the glycerin in half with water. Totally cover the herbs with the solvent. Cover with a tight fitting lid. Canning jars and lids work great for making tinctures. Let the jar sit in a warm place for 4-6 weeks. Shake the jar at least once a day.

Strain the herbs from the solvent. Just as with infused oil cover a colander with cheesecloth or linen, set on a pot and pour tincture into colander. Separate the two as much as possible. Store tinctures in a brown bottle. This prevents sunlight from breaking down the constituents.

I prefer to use fresh herbs for tinctures as the essence of the plant is really captured. I try to add the herbs in the solvent within twenty-minutes of harvesting. Most of the alcohol will dissipate if you put the drops of tincture you would like to ingest in very hot water. When I was first learning herbalism, I bought tinctures and then worked at matching the color and taste.

Compress

Compresses are cloths that have been soaked in an infusion. After squeezing out the excess fluid the cloth can then be placed on the body either hot, cold, or at room temperature.

Poultice

Poultices are similar to compresses except that the actual plant part is bruised and then put on the body. Usually a thin layer of cloth is placed on the body first and then the plant. This avoids possible irritation of the skin.

Herbal Baths

During an herbal bath the essence of the plant is absorbed through the pores of the skin. Make a strong infusion, strain and pour it in the bathtub.

Capsules

I am not a fan of capsules because so much of the sensory experienced is missed when using herbs in this form. I think it is important to smell and taste the herbs. For me the sensual experience adds in a large way to the healing process. If you prefer to use capsules buy empty ones and fill them yourself. You can powder dried herbs by grinding them in a coffee bean grinder.

The following are remedies that can be useful for common discomforts of pregnancy.

Anemia

For iron deficient anemia

- ♥ Herbs

    2 parts yellow dock root

    1 part nettles

    1 part alfalfa

    1 part dandelion root

    Preparation: Decoction/infusion, tincture

- ♥ Use cast iron skillets.

- ♥ Eat copious amounts of iron rich foods such as kale, spinach, i.e. any dark green leafy vegetables, raisins, prunes.

- ♥ Blackstrap molasses—one tablespoon three times daily— morning, noon, and evening

Back Ache

- ♥ First and foremost-keep moving and stretching—don't stay in one place too long.

- ♥ Exercises such as gardening, swimming, or yoga all keep muscles fluid.

- ♥ Massage St. John's Wort oil, or Arnica oil on sore area.

♥ Put two or three drops of peppermint or camphor essential oil in two tablespoons of olive oil and rub on sore spot.

♥ Does emotional stress settle in your back muscles? Common areas where stress collects are the neck, in the middle of the scapula, and the sacrum. Strive to understand when and why the stress settles there. Eliminate the stress if possible.

♥ Have your partner or a good friend do energy work by rubbing his/her hands together briskly, and then place his/her hands ever so gently on the sore area. Your partner may feel warmth or a tingly feeling and should maintain the hand placement until the feeling subsides. This usually takes a few minutes. You may also feel a tingly feeling or warmth. Imagine the congested energy mellowing and the pain dissipating.

♥ Pay attention to body mechanics: how are you lifting things, do you carry heavier loads on one side of your body or switch sides?

♥ Place a pillow between your legs when sleeping on your side.

♥ Visit your massage therapist, chiropractor, or acupuncturist when needed.

Colds

♥ At first sign of a cold or flu start taking Echinacea tincture and drink an Echinacea infusion.

♥ Eat raw garlic.

Sore Throat

♥ Herbs

1 part marshmallow root

1 part peppermint

Sip throughout the day

Preparation: Infusion

♥ Gargle with Echinacea tincture.

♥ Gargle with warm salt water.

Steam Inhalation with Herbs

♥ Place a handful of yarrow and peppermint leaves in a bowl and pour bowling water over them. Put face over bowl and cover head with a towel creating a tent. Breathe deeply. This remedy will make thick mucous more watery, and allow it to flow. Have a handkerchief with you!

Steam Inhalation with Essential Oils

♥ Place two to four drops of either eucalyptus, peppermint, thyme or rosemary essential oils into a bowl of just boiled water. Place face over bowl and cover with towel. Breathe deeply. Make sure you keep your eyes closed.

Cough Remedy

♥ Make a strong infusion of fresh or dried thyme (cover pot while steeping so volatile oils are not lost), mix 4 parts infusion with 2 parts honey and 1 part lemon juice. Take one teaspoon full when needed. This remedy will keep in the refrigerator for several weeks, or you can freeze it.

Herbal Bath for Colds

♥ Make a strong infusion of yarrow and thyme. Strain and place in warm bath.

Constipation

♥ **Herbs**

2 parts yellow dock root

2 parts dandelion root

1 part psyllium seeds

Preparation: Decoction/tincture

♥ Drink prune juice or eat prunes

♥ Drink more water!

♥ Massage the large intestine—the large intestine ascends on the right, moves transversely below the ribs and descends on the left. Massage clockwise.

♥ Check in with yourself emotionally. Do you feel disgust surrounding elimination? Sometimes there are long seated issues going back to potty training. Shame of the "unclean and impure" human body unfortunately can keep people from freely eliminating.

♥ Place your feet on a stool about eight to ten inches high when sitting on the toilet. This helps to move the pelvis in a different position, aiding elimination.

♥ Exercise can help, especially squatting.

Cystitis

♥ **Herbs**

1 part uva-ursi

1 part yarrow

Mix with unsweetened cranberry infusion, or make a strong cranberry infusion.

Drink one cup every four hours until symptoms have subsided.

Preparation: Infusion/tincture

Dizziness

♥ When lying down rise up slowly.

♥ Keep cool in hot weather.

♥ Eat several small meals during the day—keep your blood sugar even.

♥ Drink 2-3 quarts of water/clear liquids each day.

Heartburn

♥ Herbs

2 parts comfrey leaf

2 parts marshmallow root

1 part calendula flowers

Preparation: Infusion

♥ Is there a certain food that gives you heartburn? Avoid that food.

Eat smaller amounts at a time.

♥ Liquid dairy products such as milk, yogurt or kefir can sometimes soothe heartburn.

♥ Stay upright for a while after eating.

♥ Drink most of your daily liquids separate from meals. This will facilitate digestion by not diluting your digestive enzymes.

Hemorrhoids

♥ **Herbs**

Poultice—bruise a large plantain leaf and place on hemorrhoid for several hours.

Salve—combine plantain, yarrow, calendula. Apply to hemorrhoid.

Compress—saturate a gauze pad with a strong infusion of plantain, yarrow, calendula. Apply to hemorrhoid for several hours.

♥ Push hemorrhoid back up.

♥ Kegel—This is an exercise where you squeeze the sphincter muscles around your vagina and anus. This strengthens the muscle tone of the sphincters. Do this tightening and relaxing at least one hundred times per day.

♥ Avoid straining when eliminating—Breathe it out!

High Blood Pressure

♥ **Herbs**

2 parts hawthorn berries

2 parts motherwort

1 part garlic

Preparation: Decoction/Infusion, tincture

♥ Regular exercise can lower blood pressure.

♥ Swim.

♥ Regular massage can also lower blood pressure.

♥ Is there an emotional issue in your life that makes your blood boil? Do you have pressure in your life that is building? What can you do to lessen these issues?

♥ Be sure you are eating a high protein, whole foods diet.

♥ Avoid caffeine—drink herb teas instead (avoid green tea which has a fair amount of caffeine).

Insomnia

♥ **Herbs**

Chamomile, catnip, or valerian infusion can calm the nervou

♥ Take a warm bath with lavender before bedtime.

♥ Inhale lavender essential oil any time you want to calm the nervous system—put a drop or two on your pillow case.

♥ Drink some warm milk.

♥ Have your partner gently massage your scalp.

♥ Do you wake up at night with your mind racing and feeling worried? Train your mind to go to your favorite, real or imagined, peaceful place. Perhaps a beach or the woods, or your sacred spot mentioned in an earlier chapter. Listen to the sound of nature and let your mind relax.

Itchy Skin

♥ **Herbs**

1 part calendula flowers

1 part plantain leaves

Infuse in olive oil and cocoa butter

Rub on itchy area

♥ Oatmeal paste—Grind up oats and make a paste with water. Rub on itchy area. You can also take a bath in an oatmeal infusion.

Morning Queasiness and Vomiting

♥ **Herbs**

2 parts peppermint

1 part catnip

1 part red raspberry leaf

Preparation: Infusion, tincture

♥ Chew on candied ginger or drink ginger tea. Here's a recipe for home made ginger ale—make a decoction of fresh ginger, add honey to taste, and then add sparkling water. Adjust amounts to personal taste.

♥ Breathe deeply when a wave of nausea comes over you.

Muscle Cramps

♥ **Herbs**

2 parts alfalfa

2 parts nettle

1 part red raspberry leaf

1 part comfrey leaf

Preparation: Infusion, tincture

Drink throughout the day.

♥ Eat foods high in calcium and minerals.

♥ Exercise and stretch daily.

♥ During a cramp have your partner or good friend put their hands over the cramp until it calms. Then gently massage the crampy area. Easy going on the massage, though. You don't want the sensitive tissue to flare up again. Never massage varicose veins. You wouldn't want to accidentally dislodge a blood clot that may be held in the vein.

Nerve Calming

♥ **Herbs**

2 parts motherwort

1 part catnip

-or-

2 parts motherwort

1 part valerian

Preparation: Infusion, tincture

♥ Sit quietly in nature.

♥ Exercise daily.

♥ Massage—especially the hands and feet or have partner or friend place hands gently on any areas of tension. Breathe deeply while lying silently and imagining stress and tension melting away.

Nourish and Nurture Tea

♥ **Herbs**

Equal parts:

Red raspberry leaf

Nettles

Alfalfa

Red Clover

Preparation: Infusion

This tea is high in minerals and vitamins. Red raspberry has a special affinity for the uterus. Make a quart of this tea in the morning and drink throughout ʼthe day.

Pre-Eclampsia

♥ **Herbs**

3 parts dandelion leaf

2 parts nettles

2 part yellow dock root

1 part red raspberry

Preparation: Decoction/Infusion, tincture

♥ A high protein, nutrient dense diet is essential. Cut out any processed foods.

♥ Swim to help maintain fluid balance and edema.

♥ Drink at least 2-3 quarts of fluids per day including Nourish and Nurture tea.

Granny Janny Famous Green Goop

---

2 parts comfrey root

2 parts comfrey leaf

1 part calendula flowers

1 part plantain

Infuse all of above in olive oil.

Add 1/4 cup of grated beeswax to one cup of warm infused oil. If you are not sensitive to wool add a tablespoon of lanolin in the warmed oil also.

Preparation: Salve

I first made this salve in 1981 after the birth of my first baby. It can be used for cuts, scrapes, burns, diaper rash, sore nipples, itchy skin, razor burns; try on any skin problem.

Dosages

When thinking about dosages of herbs consider body size, and the general constitution of the person taking the herbs. The constitution of a person takes into account the person's strength, general health, vitality, and sensitivity to the environment. It is best to begin with a small amount of the herbs to see how your body reacts. Herbs such as red raspberry, nettles, red clover, and alfalfa are nourishing tonics. They are safe to use every day during pregnancy.

...Keep in mind the impact herbal remedies may have on the unborn child of a pregnant woman. The placental barrier is designed to allow nutrients to pass on to the fetus and help protect the baby from harmful substances. However, this placental barrier is permeable to many substances... Herbs such as raspberry, nettle and red clover are best suited during this time (LowDog, p.3:16).

Other herbs mentioned in this chapter are herbs of moderate strength and should be used for the ailments mentioned and not as general nutritive daily tonics. However, all are safe to use throughout your seasons of pregnancy; just not for everyday nourishment. If in doubt, find an herbalist or midwife who is experienced with herbs to guide you into mindful herbalism.

As you become more experienced, your intuitive skills will guide you when choosing herbs and deciding on their proper dosage. Listen to the body and trust its inner wisdom. Watch for signs that tell you what and how much the body needs. In general, infusions and decoctions use 1 to 3 tablespoons of fresh herb or root, or 1 to 3 teaspoons of dried, per six-eight ounces of water. Tinctures are from 1/4 to 1 teaspoon three times daily.

Remember that taking herbs is not like taking a prescription pill.

The following dosage chart comes from Rosemary Gladstar's lovely book, *Family Herbal: A Guide to Living Life With Energy, Health, and Vitality.*

Adult Dosages

Chronic problems are long-term imbalances such as hay fever, arthritis, back pain, insomnia, and long-standing bronchial problems. Chronic problems can, however, flare up with acute symptoms. Follow these guidelines for treating chronic problems.

Tea: 3 to 4 cups daily for several weeks

Tinctures: 1/2 to 1 teaspoon three times daily

Capsules: 2 capsules three times daily

Acute Problems are sudden, reaching a crisis and needing quick attention. Examples of acute problems include toothaches, migraines, bleeding, burns, and sudden onset of cold or flu. Follow these guidelines for treating acute health problems.

Tea: 1/4 to 1/2 cup served throughout the day, up to 3 to 4 cups

Tinctures: 1/4 to 1/2 teaspoon every 30 to 60 minutes (Gladstar, 2001, p. 379).

Keep in mind that although the natural remedies discussed in this chapter are gentle; all of them may have powerful effects on the body. However, don't expect to always see instant results. Sometimes massaged muscles don't release for hours afterwards. Tonic herbs may have a cumulative effect on overall health. Exercise, sunshine, and fresh air most likely will lighten the spirit for hours afterwards. Pay attention to the inner workings of your body and the inner togetherness of motherbaby.

~Thirteen~

Continuing the Journey

Peace begins at birth. A natural mother intuitively knows that it does matter, not only for the baby, but also for the mother herself, how a baby is born. A gentle loving birth, from a mother well cared for and nurtured, is the beginning of a peaceful understanding and existence of life on this earth. Birth activist and author, Suzanne Arms, wrote this profound poem,

A Hand Full of Hope
If we hope to create
a non-violent world
where respect and kindness
replace fear and hatred,
we must begin
with how we treat each other
at the beginning of life.

For that is where
our deepest patterns are set.
From these roots
grow fear and alienation
~or love and trust.
© Suzanne Arms, Birthing The Future ®

Of course, babies come into this world as their own person, with the story of their life ready to be played out. This baby, this unique individual, came to be cared for by you. Why, at this time in world history, did this baby, your baby, come to be born? Why are you the mother of this new person and not another? Did your baby choose you to be his/her mother? In the greater scheme of life these questions are too enormous to even begin to understand, but are much-needed questions to explore.

Following a natural mothering path, the less worn path, is honoring all of those who have gone before you. It involves reaching into your cellular memories and remembering all of the mothers from the past. Our tissues are made from our ancestors. While listening to our inner wisdom we are remembering their joys and pains and gathering their knowledge. Throughout your seasons of pregnancy, the journey of birth, and motherbaby moon time you are gathering information from the past, and creating a new future, while living in the moment. You truly are the divine feminine energy, the embodied female.

You are giving a great gift to the world, to your baby and to yourself, by the fact that you, as a vessel for new life, are willing to go towards the depth of your being to be a natural mother. You are willing to follow a path that you alone must journey. Through living your convictions you are not asking a midwife or doctor to rescue you, or asking your attendant to make the labor and birth process happen without feeling it. You are willing to feel it all!

This is not to say that if your birth story doesn't end the way you planned that you will be forever unhappy. Remember that every story teaches us about life, and ourselves in general. Learn what you can from each experience and focus on the many layers of possibilities. Sometimes things happen for a reason that we may never understand.

As you begin the awesome task of cultivating and nurturing your baby, look back to all that you have learned throughout your seasons of pregnancy, journey of birth, and motherbaby moon time. Indeed, much of what you have learned during the past four seasons will guide you on the next chapter of your life together as a family.

We'll leave the last words to this ancient Chinese text:

What is well planted cannot be uprooted.
What is well embraced cannot slip away.
Your descendants will carry on the ancestral
sacrifice for generations without end.
Cultivate virtue in your own person,
And it becomes a genuine part of you.
Cultivate it in the family,

And it will abide.

Cultivate it in the community,

And it will grow.

Cultivate it in the state,

And it will flourish abundantly.

Cultivate it in the world,

And it will be universal.

Hence, a person must be judged as person;

A family as family;

A community as community;

A state as a state;

And the world as world.

How do I know about the world?

By what is within me.

—Lao Tzu

As you continue on your voyage I hope that you delve deeply into life's mysteries. Caring for this new baby is the most important work you will ever do. Blessings on your journey!

References

Arms, S. (2004), *A Hand Full of Hope* from *Birthing The Future Website,* Retrieved on 02/06/2005 from http://www.BirthingThe Future.com/.

Balch, J., & Balch P. (1997). *Prescription for nutritional healing.* Garden City Park, New York: Avery Publishing Group.

Chaitow, L. (1999). *Hydrotherapy: water therapy for health & beauty.* Boston: Element Books.

Cohen, J. (1999). Why Homebirth? Originally published *Midwifery Today,* Issue 50, Summer, 1999. Retrieved 08/25/2004 from http://www.midwiferytoday.com.

Davies, L. (2001). Having a Baby is Like Running a Marathon Because ... Originally published in *The Practicing Midwife,* Retrieved 08/23/2004 from http://www.withwoman.co.uk.

Davis, E. (1997). *Heart and hands: a midwife's guide to pregnancy & birth.* Berkeley, CA: Celestial Arts.

Davis-Floyd, R. (1992). *Birth as an American rite of passage.* Berkeley, CA: University of California Press.

de Bairacli-Levy, J. (1971). *Nature's children: a guide to organic foods and herbal remedies for children.* New York: Schocken Books.

Dunham, C. (1991). *Mamatoto: a celebration of birth.* New York: Penguin Books.

Durbin, B. (2004). Delicious Color. *Newhouse News Service.* Kalamazoo Gazette, April 19, 2004.

Ecclesiates, 3:1. (King James Version).

Emoto, M. (2004). *The hidden messages in water.* Hillsboro, Oregon; Beyond Words Books.

Fischer-Rizzi, A. (1990). *Complete aromatherapy handbook: essential oils for radiant health.* New York: Sterling.

Frye, A. (1995). *Holistic Midwifery: volume I care during pregnancy.* Portland, Oregon: Labrys Press.

Frye, A. (1997). *Understanding diagnostic tests in the childbearing year.* (6th ed.). Portland, Oregon: Labrys Press.

Gladstar, R. (2001). *Family herbal: a guide to living life with energy, health, and vitality.* North Adams, Massachusetts: Storey Books.

Global Vaccine Institute. (2004). *Immunization ploys: Are parents being manipulated?* Retrieved 08/18/2004 from http://thinktwice.com.

Incao M.D., P. (1999). *How vaccinations work: will this unorthodox view gain serious consideration?* Personal correspondance, Retrieved 08/18/2004 from www.garynull.com.

Hood, E. (2003). Organic food for thought: Lessening children's pesticide exposure. *Environmental Health Perspectives.* 111, no3, A166, March 2003.

Johnson, C. (1997). *Cooking like a goddess; bringing seasonal magic into the kitchen.* Rochester, Vermont: Healing Arts Press.

Kaptchuk, T. (1983). *The web that has no weaver: understanding Chinese medicine.* Chicago: Congdon & Weed.

Kimmel, J. (2003). *The nurturing mother.* Retrieved 07/22/2003 from www.naturalchild.org.

Kirschmann, J. (1996). *Nutrition almanac.* New York; McGraw-Hill.

Kitzinger, S. (2000). *Rediscovering birth.* New York: Simon & Schuster.

La Leche League, (2004,). *The womanly art of breastfeeding.* (7th ed.). Franklin Park, Illinois: La Leche League.

Low Dog, T. (1996). *Foundations in herbal medicine correspondance course.* (Available from Foundations in Herbal Medicine, 112 Hermosa, Albuquerque NM 87108).

Luce, J. (2004). The knowing body and remembering heart. *Midwifery Today.* Issue 69, Spring 2004, p. 19.

McCarty, W. (1999). *Being with babies: what babies are teaching us.* (1996). Goleta, California: Wondrous Beginnings. http://www.BeingwithBabies.com.

Monte, T. (1993). *World medicine: the east west guide to healing your body.* New Your: Tarcher/Perigee.

Myss, C. (1996). *Anatomy of the spirit: the seven stages of power and healing.* New York: Random House.

Northrup, C. (1994). *Women's bodies, women's wisdom: creating physical and emotional health and healing.* New York: Bantam Books.

Odent, M. (2002). *The farmer and the obstetrician.* London; Free Association Books.

Odent, M. (1999). *The scientification of love.* London; Free Association Books.

Paul-Bort, D. (Executive Producer). (1999). *Birth day.* [Video]. United States: Sage Femme, Inc. (Available from http://www.homebirthvideos.com).

Pert, C. (1997). *Molecules of emotion.* New York: Scribner.

Phillips, M., & Phillips, N. (2001). *The village herbalist: sharing plant medicines with family and community.* White River Junction, VT; Chelsea Green Publishing.

Pickering, W. (2004). *Make health your priority! You deserve it!* Retrieved March 25, 2004 from http://www.allnatural.com

Ray, M. (1997). *Eighty two percent of the world's men are intact.* Retrieved on 08/22/2004 from http://www.cirp.org.

Reagan, L. (2001). Show Us the Science: An Exclusive Mothering Report on the Second International Public Conference of the National Vaccine Information Center. *Mothering Magazine.* Issue 105. March/April.

Reeves, P. (1999). *Women's intuition: unlocking the wisdom of the body.* Berkeley, California: Conari Press.

Schwartz, F. (1997). Music and perinatal stress reduction. *Prenatal and Perinatal Psychology and Health.* 12(1), Fall.

Sears, J. (2001). Mangia, Mama! *Baby Talk.* 66, no7, p.46-50, Spring 2001.

Spintage, R. & Droh, R. (1987). *Effects of anxioloytic music on plasma levels of stress hormones in different medical specialites.* The fourth international symposium on music: Rehabilitation and human well-being (pp. 88-101). Lanham, MD: University Press of America.

Soloman, G. (2001). *Healthy milk, healthy baby.* Retrieved 08/23/2004 from http://www.nrdc.org.

Starhawk. (2004). *The earth path: grounding your spirit in the rhythms of nature.* New York: Harper Collins.

Sullivan, K. (1998). *The healing power of touch: the many ways physical contact can cure.* Lincolnwood, IL: Publictions International.

Tamaro, J. (1996). *So that's what they are for: breastfeeding basics.* Boston: Adams Publishing.

Tzu, L. Translated by Wu, J. (1961). *Tao Teh Ching.*
New York: St. John's University Press.

Vaughan, F. (1998). *Awakening Intuition.* Thinking
Allowed: Conversations on the Leading Edge of
Knowledge and Discovery with Dr. Jeffrey Mishlove.
Retrieved 07/29/2003 from http://www.intuition.org.

www.diet-and-health.net. (2004). Retrieved 06/23/2004

Weed, S. (1989). *Wise woman herbal: healing wise.*
Woodstock, NY: Ash Tree Publishing.

Wickham, S. (2004). *Sacred cycles: the spirals of
women's well being.* London: Free Association
Books.

Wickham, S. (2002). *What's right for me? Making
decisions in pregnancy and birth.* London: AIMS.

Williamson, M. (1999). *Enchanted love: The mystical
power of intimate relationships.* New York: Simon &
Schuster.

Worthington, V. (2003). *Organic produce is better for
you. R*etrieved 03/03/2004 from
http://www.organicgardening.com.

For Further Reading

The Seasons of Pregnancy

Arms, S. (1994). *Immaculate deception II: a fresh look at childbirth*. Berkeley, CA: Celestial Arts.

Baker, J., Baker, F., Slayton, T. (1986). *Conscious conception: elemental journey through the labyrinth of sexuality*. Monroe, UT: Freestone.

Baldwin, R. (1995). *Special delivery*. Berkeley, CA: Celestial Arts.

Cohen, N., Estner, L. (1983). *Silent knife*. South Hadley, MA: Bergin & Garvey.

Cohen, N. (1991). *Open season: a survival guide for natural childbirth and VBAC in the '90s*. Westport, CT: Bergin & Garvey.

England, P., Horowitz, R. (1998). *Birthing from within: an extra-ordinary guide to childbirth preparation*. Albuquerque, NM: Partera Press.

Freedom, L. (1999). *Birth as a healing experience: the emotional journey of pregnancy through postpartum*. Binghamtom, NY: Harrington Park Press.

Goer, H. (1995). *Obstetric myths versus research realities: a guide to the medical literature*. Westport, CT: Bergin & Garvey.

Harper-Roth, J. (2001). *The pregnancy herbal: holistic remedies, nutritional therapies, and soothing treatments from nature's pharmacy for the mother-to-be*. New York: Three Rivers Press.

Kitzinger, S. (1996). *The complete book of pregnancy and childbirth*. New York: Alfred A. Knopf.

Nilsson, L. (1990). *A child is born*. New York: Delacorte Press.

O'Mara, P. (2003). *Having a baby, naturally*. New York: Atria Books.

Sears, M., Sears, W. (1997). *The pregnancy book: a month-by-month guide*. Boston: Little Brown.

Steingraber, S. (2001). *Having faith: an ecologist's journey to motherhood*. Cambridge, MA: Perseus.

Journey of Birth

Baldwin, R. (1995). *Special delivery*. Berkeley, CA: Celestial Arts.

Gaskin, I. (1990). *Spiritual midwifery*. 3d ed. Summertown, TN: Book Publishing Company.

Kitzinger, S. (1992). *Being born*. Rutherford, NJ: Berkeley.

Kitzinger, S. (1989). *Giving birth: how it really feels*. New York: Farrar, Straus, and Biroux.

Simkin, P. (1989). *The birth partner: everything you need to know to help a woman through childbirth.* Boston: Harvard Common Press.

Motherbaby Moon Time

Adamson, E., Kays, M. (1999). *Breastfeeding: a holistic handbook.* New York: Berkeley.

Bing, E., Colman, L. (1997). *Laughter and tears: a complete guide to the emotional life of new mothers.* New York: Henry Holt.

Bossi, L., Gosline, A., (1999). *Mother's nature: timeless wisdom for the journey into motherhood.* Berkeley, CA: Conari Press.

Kitzinger, S. (1994). *The year after childbirth.* New York: Fireside Books.

Kitzinger, S. (1998). *Breastfeeding your baby.* Rev. ed. New York:Knopf.

La Leche League Inernational. (1997). *The womanly art of breastfeeding.* New York: Plume.

Lim, R. (2001). *After the baby's birth, a woman's way to wellness: a complete guide for postpartum women.* Rev. ed. Berkeley, CA: Celestial Arts.

Miller, N. (2002). *Vaccines: are they really safe and effective?* Sante Fe, NM: New Atlantean Press.

Odent, M. (1992). *The nature of birth and breastfeeding.* Westport, CT: Bergin & Barvey.

Placksin, S. (2000). *Mothering the new mother: women's feelings and needs after childbirth*. New York: Newmarket Press.

Sears, M., Sears, W. (2000). *The breastfeeding book: everything you need to know about nursing your child from birth through weaning*. New York: Little, Brown.

O'Mara, P., ed. (1993). *Circumcision: the rest of the story—a selection of articles, letters, and resources*. Sante Fe, NM: Mothering.

Ritter, T. (2002). *Doctors re-examine circumcision*. Hurricane, WV: Third Millenium.

Romm, A.J. (2001). *Vaccinations: a thoughtful parent's guide—how to make safe, sensible decisions about the risks, benefits and alternatives*. Rochester, VT: Healing Arts Press.

Web Sites Focused on Natural Mothering

www.askdrsears.com
www.birthpartners.com
www.childbirth.org
www.compleatmother.com
www.creativebirthingarts.com
www.diaperpin.com
www.mothering.com
www.naturalchild.com

www.life.ca
www.praireinet.org
www.rebozoway.com
www.withwoman.co.uk
www.midwifeinfo.com
www.light-hearts.com
www.gentlebirth.org
www.midwiferytoday.com

For herbal products and herbal support contact:
Granny Janny Herbs
12901 Fort Custer Drive
Galesburg, MI 49053
(269) 665-7797
www.creativebirthingarts.com

Index

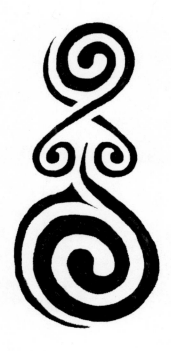

© Allison McKenna